CONTENTS

· ·

Dedication

I dedicate this book to my dad who suffered from and succumbed to heart disease at the age of 71. His death caused me to embark on a journey to seek a healthier life. Thanks, dad, for your ultimate sacrifice. I miss you every day.

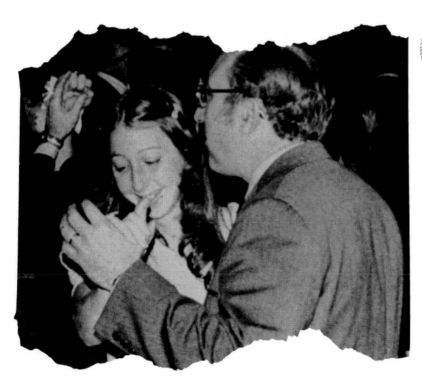

Acknowledgments

While the spiritual inspiration and drive to writing this book came from my Dad, the continued journey and final efforts were driven by several key individuals. First, I want to thank my dear friend Nancy who is the original vegan and helped me so much in the early days of my journey and is my biggest cheerleader. I am thankful for my friends Mike and Cheryl who encouraged me by their amazing transformations via a WFPB diet to begin teaching this way of living to others. Of course, I need to thank my good friend Don. I think if it wasn't for our mutual efforts in writing our first books and our endless discussions and cheering each other on throughout the process, I would never have come this far. He finished his race and was there rallying for me to finish mine. I have to thank my Wellness20 partner Brooke Ali for getting me to the finish line with her inspiration, wise counsel, and dedication to furthering the health and wellness of the planet. She inspires me every day. To my husband Travis who has been with me through all of the ups and downs, and supports and encourages me in my life's pursuits, no matter how big or small. He is truly my life partner. Finally, to my three beautiful children, you are the moon, stars, and universe to me.

Introduction

Life is a journey, filled with twists and turns where we find the expected and unexpected. Years ago I took a journey to reclaim my health with no idea of what lay ahead. With the simple purchase of one book, the world of true health was revealed to me. Then began an avalanche of information gathering, reading everything I could get my hands on, enrolling in nutrition courses, career changes, and teaching what I had learned to others. To say that I was driven to write this book would be fair. I could not keep this in me if I tried. I wrote this book in a simple and colorful way so that anyone beginning this journey would not be turned off by the change that is involved in taking charge of your health. WFPB20 (an acronym for whole food, plant-based) is not a treatise on nutrition but simply a lifestyle plan and a step-by-step guide to the why and how of adopting a healthy lifestyle. It's the kind of information that I would have wanted to have when I first began my journey. There is still so much for all of us to learn, which in my opinion makes life more interesting. I hope this book will help you wherever you are on your journey to get you to the next junction on the road to health and wellness.

For me personally, I am most moved when I hear someone else's story on how they took back their health and fought for the quality of life they deserved. This is true empowerment. Two women who have inspired me along the way have shared their stories for you in my book. I hope that they inspire you as well. Wishing you a wonderful journey through WFPB20.

BROOKE ALI went vegan to feel better. She had been feeling lethargic, achy, and had IBD issues. Going vegan helped tremendously. She lost weight, felt younger, and had more clarity. However, as her journey continued, those same health issues began to return along with additional issues. She decided to clean up her diet by going completely whole food plant-based, but that still wasn't enough. Her next step was to cut out gluten from her diet and that seemed to help. However, when she tried having it again, her symptoms came back even stronger, to the point of great depression and extreme pain in all of her joints, blurry eyesight, and IBS.

Brooke was diagnosed with Hashimoto's disease and Hypothyroidism and ended up going on medication for Hypothyroidism and depression. The medication helped some but came with many undesirable side effects. She was determined to find the root of the problem, so she began studying macrobiotics and juicing.

Through a combination of adding iodine, celery juicing, and cutting out nightshade vegetables and gluten, she was able to go off of her medications and heal. It was a long and slow journey, but she learned to listen to her body and apply a lot of self-care rituals as well. She still continues to learn and discover new things. Such as how sugar triggers inflammation and how easy it is to stray from the healthful way of eating. She has devoted her life to sharing her story and recipes with others.

She has now partnered with Patricia Thomson in their business venture Wellness20 and has contributed her expertise in the recipes found here in WFPB20.

DENISE woke up one morning unable to move her body. Thinking she had had a stroke, her family rushed her to the ER where after multiple tests and blood work, she was diagnosed with severe Rheumatoid Arthritis (RA). RA is an autoimmune disease where your own immune system begins to attack your body's tissues and joints causing severe inflammation, bone erosion and deformity, and pain. Denise was immediately put on methotrexate, which is a strong cancer drug with serious side effects, to suppress her immune system. She could not walk, get dressed and at times, could not even get out of bed. The doctors told her that she would be this way for the rest of her life, but she knew there had to be a better way. She started doing research on her own and began cutting out dairy, processed foods, and sugar. She started to feel a little better, but it was still not a complete success. Denise was frustrated. The last straw came when the newest drug she was on put her at risk of heart failure. At that point, she decided to go off all of her medications and work on a more natural solution. After much research, she adopted a whole-food, plant-based lifestyle, and within 3 months she went into complete remission from her RA. She now functions as if she never had RA. No joint pain, sleeps normally, and lives a fully functional, high-quality life where she can now enjoy the love of her family and friends.

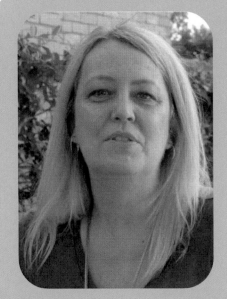

Chapter One

THE JOURNEY

The Skinny on the WFPB20 Lifestyle Plan

Welcome to WFPB20! Imagine a way of eating that encourages you to eat a variety of foods that are not only nutritious but great tasting. Your health will improve, your body will change, and you will begin to feel more energy and an overall better feeling of being. Like a rainbow, this life plan will include natural foods representing every color of the spectrum. It is a whole-food, plant-based (WFPB) way of eating that includes foods found in nature that are from minimally processed ingredients.

If you are reading this book, chances are you have come to a point in your life where you would like to make changes—whether it is due to health issues, a desire to lose weight, or as the result of something that has happened or is happening in your life. You have come to the right place.

This book is not based on gimmicks or extremes. With the exception of your weekly groceries (you may actually see cost savings), you won't have to buy additional supplements, equipment, or pay monthly fees to eat this way. The world of whole food is yours to explore.

WFPB20 is really about awareness, empowerment, and encouragement.

WFPB20 is really about awareness, empowerment, and encouragement. There is no judgment, guilt, or ridicule. Everyone has to travel their health journey at their pace. This is why so many diets do not work. It is either their way or the highway. If you read and absorb the information that is shared in this book, you will suddenly see things differently and in their true form and meaning.

Once you know and understand all that you will read here, you will not be able to erase it from your mind. It is the hope that you will want to share your newfound knowledge with others who could benefit. Don't think of this as something you have to do for the rest of your life. Just dip your toe in for 20 days and see how it feels. Believe that at the end of the 20 days you will be in a totally different mindset from where you are right now. Sometimes it is better not to eat the whole enchilada at once but to savor each and every bite and revel in the flavors as they reveal themselves to you. You are encouraged to embrace WFPB20 and take one day at a time. Explore how you feel, embrace the newness, and enjoy this wonderful journey to better health that you are on. And yes, enchiladas are on the menu!

One of the first considerations of adopting WFPB20 is understanding that it does not include animal products of any kind, i.e. no dairy, eggs, fish, animal flesh or any products derived from animals such as bovine extracts, bone broth, or gelatins. It is a plant-based approach to food. This may bring up many questions in your mind. This book will take you step by step and explain what it is exactly that you will be eating, why you should be eating this way, how you will prepare your meals, how you will shop for your food, how you will eat out, on the road tips, establishing new family traditions, and how to navigate all of the temptations, bumps, and detours in the healthy road ahead. In addition, this book will provide you with the rationale for this seemingly crazy omission of a basic food source for most people.

Secondly, this book is not about adopting a diet but rather a lifestyle. Even though it is introduced as a 20-day experience, you won't want to do this for the short term. Over those 20 days, you will soon realize that you want to do this for the long term. Prove me wrong but I think you will have a hard time giving this all up at the end of the 20 days.

> This book is not about adopting a diet but rather a lifestyle.

So what does plant-based mean? It means you can still eat pizza, pasta, sandwiches, wraps, stir fry, burgers, hot dogs, potatoes, tacos, rice and noodle bowls, pancakes, French toast, breakfast scrambles, refried beans, lasagna, soups, chilis, gravies, sauces, smoothies, cakes, cookies, and frozen desserts, to name a few. You can eat from a variety of cuisines such as Asian, Italian, French, Cuban, Mexican, Mediterranean, Indian,

Southern, Southwestern, or simple American fare. That is an incredible list of foods, right? Sounds like some of the foods you have been eating all along. The difference lies in the fact that all of these foods can be prepared with plant-based ingredients. There is no reason to add unhealthy ingredients if you can still have the same wonderful enjoyment of eating these foods. Doesn't that make sense?

> By adding plant-based foods to your plate you leave less and less room for unhealthy foods.

Think of this way of eating as the "replacement plan." Basically, you are replacing unhealthy foods with healthy foods. By adding plant-based foods to your plate, you leave less and less room for unhealthy foods. Before you know it, your plate is filled with delicious healthy foods and you begin to not miss the "old" foods.

WFPB20 is set up in a 20-day cycle with easy to follow and prepare recipes, colorful photos, and grocery lists. Plus, loaded with tips, shopping guides, nutrition information, resources, and scientific sources, you will have all of the tools you need to move forward in a successful and healthy way.

You will learn a whole new way of food preparation, but this does not mean you will spend all of your time in the kitchen. Recipes can be quick and easy or more involved depending on how much time you want to spend. Plus, most of the ingredients you will need for the first 20 days are pretty basic. You can get fancier if you want to once you feel more comfortable eating and cooking this way.

The Standard American Diet (SAD)

In order to understand what this book is about, you will need to first understand what our current state of eating is in our families, cultures, local communities, countries, and the world. You can't move in a new direction if you don't understand where you are starting from. This will hopefully provide some motivation to keep on this journey.

The Standard American Diet (SAD) consists of fast fried foods, processed foods, meats, eggs, sugar, salt, dairy, and oils. Vegetables, fruit, and whole grains are low on the list. Over 75% of the US population do not follow healthy dietary guidelines. [1] It is no wonder that the acronym for the Standard American Diet is SAD.

While the SAD describes the way Americans eat, it is not limited to just the US, although Americans seem to excel in this compared to other countries.

However, it is a fact that other countries are catching up and seeing the same increased rates of disease as in the US.

> Over 75% of the US population do not follow healthy dietary guidelines.

Diseases related to our SAD lifestyle, like heart disease, cancer, diabetes, and obesity, have skyrocketed in the US and globally. It is a very sad state of affairs that most people have gotten themselves into. In addition to the immense personal toll, the SAD also has an economic impact, particularly driving up healthcare costs at unsustainable levels.[2] These diseases undermine our health, shorten our lives, and cause immeasurable pain, suffering, disability, and economic costs for everyone.

How is WFPB20 Different from Other Diets?

The concept of eating a bounty of food is very different from most other diets where you are restricted to eating certain kinds of food and limited in the quantity of food you can eat. Plus, there are diets that restrict the timing of your meals and limit the number of meals you can have. Weighing in, counting calories, counting points, and taking a bunch of supplements are all common themes to other diets. There is none of that with WFPB20. This plan is based on 20 days since it takes anywhere from 20 days to 3 months to make new habits. Think of this plan as a "Jumpstart" to get you headed in the right direction.

Nutrient-Dense vs Calorie Dense

One basic concept of WFPB20 is that you will eat a plentiful amount of plant-based foods— foods that are rich in nutrients and fiber—foods that will fill you up and nourish your body—foods that are nutrient-dense. You will move away from those calorie-dense foods—foods that are full of fat, cholesterol, hormones, antibiotics, additives—foods that don't fill you up since they lack fiber and do very little to nourish your body but rather wreak havoc on your body.

What would you rather eat?

The concept of eating a bounty of food is very different from most other diets.

6

Foods with high levels of nutrients or foods with high levels of calories? Foods that will nourish your body and help to prevent disease or foods that have been scientifically proven to cause disease like obesity, heart disease, cancer, diabetes, auto-immune diseases, Alzheimer's, and arthritis?

No Calorie Counting

It is a scientific fact that when you eat more calories than you burn, you gain weight. The opposite happens when you eat fewer calories than you burn—you guessed it you lose weight. When you consume the same number of calories in as the number of calories burned you remain at the same weight. No matter what diet or meal plan you are on, these are the basic tenets of weight loss, weight gain, and weight maintenance.

However, all calories are not the same. Consuming 100 calories of olive oil does not satiate

All calories are not the same.

you in the same way as consuming 100 calories of sweet potato. Nor does it provide the same nutritional density. There is no fiber and very little nutrients in 100 calories of olive oil. You will not feel satiated. On the other hand, potatoes are loaded with fiber, vitamins, and nutrients vital to your cells. This is so very important to understand. This is why most diets fail in the long run. The foods you are restricted to on typical diets are not filling or satiating, leading dieters to stray from their diets in search of fulfillment. This is the reason why adopting a plant-based lifestyle is so successful. The foods you eat are nutrient-dense—filling you up and satiating your hunger.

By adopting a plant-based lifestyle you will not only feel fuller, but you will be nurturing your body with nutrient-dense foods.

You can actually eat less food and feel completely satisfied. You will not need to count calories as long as you are following the basic principles of this plan— whole, plant-based foods, minimally processed.

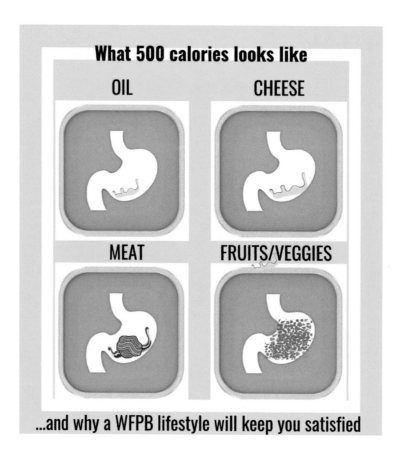

What 500 calories looks like

OIL   CHEESE

MEAT   FRUITS/VEGGIES

...and why a WFPB lifestyle will keep you satisfied

Chapter Two

EAT WHAT YOU NEED

· ·

The Main Components of WFPB20

Despite the confusing and confounding media messages we have been fed all of our lives related to our diets, fats, carbs, and proteins are the foundational building blocks of the food we need. It is the form these building blocks are in when we ingest them that truly determines our health. A whole-food, plant-based form.

We need fats, carbs, and proteins in our diet. Every day. Absolutely. Each one of these is responsible for numerous critical functions in our bodies. Diets

9

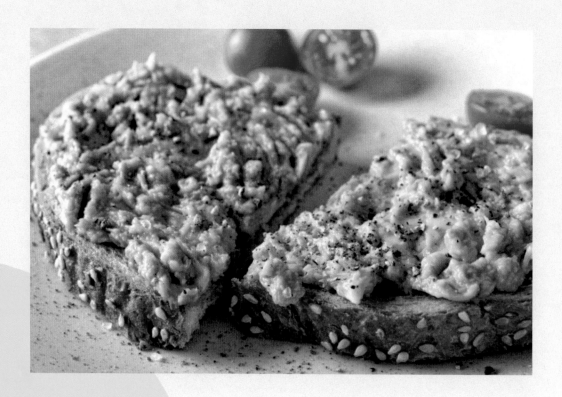

that omit any of these are built on faulty reasoning and science. WFPB20 is based on sound scientific principles as well as sound scientific research. It is essentially built around the concept of the three nutritional elements we need to consume on a daily basis. In order to understand the basic concept of this plan, we need to delve into some specifics about fats, carbs, and proteins.

Why We Need Fats

Even though we have been inundated with negative messaging around eating fats, they are vital to our health. Fats are instrumental in the absorption of several fat-soluble vitamins and nutrients such as vitamin A, D, and E. Fats provide energy for the body and are crucial in cell growth and hormone production. Fats help to protect our organs and maintain our body temperature. Our brains are composed of 50% fat, so fats play a vital role in our brain health. In addition, the fats we consume are an important source of omega-3 fatty acids. More to come on omega-3s later on in this chapter.

Fats come in all kinds of shapes and sizes as well as from different sources. Structurally, they fall into two basic categories: saturated and unsaturated. The difference lies in the single bonds found in saturated fats and the double and triple bonds found in unsaturated fats. Saturated fats tend to be less stable than unsaturated fats and are usually solid at room temperature, like coconut oil, margarine, and lard yet when heat is applied, you can melt them. The more stable unsaturated fats are mostly liquid at room temperature like avocado oil, peanut oil, and olive oil, when heated they keep their liquid form.

One type of unsaturated fat that has received a great deal of attention are trans fats. These fats can be found naturally in the guts of some animals and then end up in food products (e.g. dairy and meat) but more commonly, these fats are made

Fats provide energy for the body and are crucial in cell growth and hormone production.

commercially by transforming liquid fats into solid fats and are used in many processed foods (you may also know them as partially hydrogenated fats or oils). Trans fats have been notoriously ostracized (and rightly so) in the scientific community and in the media for wreaking havoc on our health, including increasing our risk of heart disease, diabetes and obesity. [1] [2] [3] [4] Another important point: in June 2015, the FDA stated that partially hydrogenated oils were no longer considered Generally Recognized as Safe for human health. [5]

Omega-3s

Omega-3 fatty acids are necessary for blood clotting and

help in the formation of the cell membranes in our brains. Research studies have shown that including omega-3s in your diet can lead to a decrease in cardiovascular and memory disorders. [6]

There are two main forms of omega-3 fatty acids: ALA, which is short for alpha-linolenic acid, and EPA/DHA, which is mercifully short for eicosapentaenoic acid and docosahexaenoic acid. ALA is found in plant sources such as dark leafy greens, walnuts, flax, chia, and hemp seeds. EPAs/DHAs are considered extra long-chain omega-3s and primarily found in certain fish and in algae. Provided that we are feeding our bodies whole-food that is plant-based and without processed foods and animal products, our bodies can convert short-chain ALA into these extra long-chain omega-3s without the need to consume fish. Including natural, fresh, plant-based sources of ALA such as nuts, seeds, and dark leafy greens in your diet

should ensure that your body is getting all of the omega-3s it needs. A note of caution: there have been studies indicating that we may not be efficient at at converting ALA to EPA/DHA and therefore pollutant-free algae supplements (250 mg/day) are recommended by some to ensure that we have sufficient levels of both EPA and DHA. [7] [8] [9] [10]

Which Fats Should You Avoid And Which Fats Should You Consume?

Fats can have both positive and negative effects on the body when consumed. There are healthy fats and unhealthy fats, and the choice between the two is one determining factor for your health. Eating a plate of French fries cooked in trans fat is the fast track to heart disease and a host of other ailments. Pouring olive oil on your salad or cooking with coconut oil is adding 100% pure fat to your food without adding any nutritional value. Worse, the oil is an irritant to our blood vessels, causing inflammation in its wake as it travels through the body.

Fats in their whole form, or minimally processed and rich in nutrients and fiber are your target. Packed in their natural fiber-enriched forms, they move through your system smoothly and feed your cells the fat nourishment they need. Eating avocado sliced in a salad, ground flaxseed sprinkled on your oatmeal, almond butter on your whole-grain toast, peanut butter in your African stew, or olives on your pizza are examples of how to get healthy fats into your diet.

By contrast, animal products contain lots of fat and no fiber of any kind. When you consume animal fats, not only are you ingesting the fats, but also cholesterol and other toxic substances. In addition, you are consuming all of the hormones, waste products, and chemicals that were circulating in

> ## Fats in their whole form, or minimally processed and rich in nutrients and fiber are your target.

the animal's body before it was killed. Everything that an animal has been exposed to during its life is in the meat you eat. Have you seen where commercially grown animals in the US live most of their lives?

Animal fats have been directly linked to inducing an inflammatory response in your body. Think of it like rubbing sandpaper on your skin. Your body's blood vessels are lined with a single layer of flattened endothelial cells that make up the endothelium.

The endothelium is a dynamic structure that extends throughout the body and lines every single organ and blood vessel. It has a myriad of very critical functions, such as regulating the flow of blood and the pumping of the heart; repairing blood vessels; helping to control inflammation and blood clotting; and serves as a selectively permeable barrier. The fat you put into your mouth eventually ends up being transported throughout your blood vessels. As it moves along, it is recognized as a foreign substance and thus irritates the endothelium, causing an inflammatory reaction. Inflammation is believed to be the root cause of many of our dietary-related diseases, such as heart disease, diabetes, obesity, cancer, arthritis, and auto-immune diseases. [11]

All plant-based foods contain some degree of fat. The foods with higher healthier fat content include avocados, nuts, seeds, and ground flaxseed. To minimize adverse health effects, it is best to avoid all foods with trans fats, including meat, dairy, fried, and processed foods.

It is important to note that healthy fats come with higher calorie content and a diet high in these foods without a reciprocal calorie expenditure in the form of exercise or physical activity can result in weight gain. Also, individuals with cardiovascular disease are advised to minimize their consumption of plant-based foods high in dietary fat. [12] [13]

Do These Carbs Make Me Look Fat?

People are passionate about their carbs. There is no doubt that they are the source of much debate. Do a Google search and you will find reams of sites that either support or denounce carbs. It is almost political. Heated discussions abound, sometimes very intense discussions about low carbs, high carbs, no carbs.

> All plant-based foods contain some degree of fat.

Forget all of the negative messaging you have heard about carbohydrates. We absolutely need carbohydrates to live. It is the source of the carbohydrate that is up for discussion. Carbohydrates, made up of neutral molecules of carbon, hydrogen, and oxygen, are the body's fuel source. The only natural sources of carbohydrates are plants. Whole food, plant-based carbohydrates are not only healthy for you but are essential for proper cell functioning.

When we consume a carbohydrate, its digestion begins in our mouths through enzymes in our salivary glands. It is broken down into less complex sugars and absorbed into the bloodstream in our small intestines. The basic components of a naturally occurring carbohydrate are simple sugars like glucose. Our cells live on glucose. Our brains require glucose, and only glucose, to function. Glucose is found naturally in grains, potatoes, rice, corn, legumes, vegetables, fruits, nuts,

> Whole food, plant-based carbohydrates are not only healthy for you but essential for proper cell functioning.

and seeds. Loading up on processed carbohydrates such as sugars, cereals, chips, cookies, cakes, and bread is what gets us into trouble. Our bodies have a hard time processing these foods and extracting anything nutritious for the cells to use.

A potato is filled with carbohydrates plus fiber and a whole host of nutrients. When you consume a baked potato, your body uses the components in the potato for everyday functioning. When glucose is produced from the potato your brain has food, your cells have food, your digestive system has fiber—everyone is happy. However, when you add butter, cheese, bacon bits, salt, and sour cream, everything good about the potato is negated. Now your body is busy processing all of the unhealthy fats you just poured on top of a perfectly good fuel source. The fats slow down your metabolism and you feel sluggish along with the rest of your organs. The fats clog up your cells, attach to the walls of your vessels, and load up your liver and bile ducts.

Why We Need Protein

We need protein to live, however, not to the extent that the meat and dairy industry, the media, and others would have us consume it. Plus, the form of protein that you put into your body makes all of the difference in the world. We are a country obsessed with getting enough protein, yet is is rare that physicians in the US treat anyone with a serious protein deficiency. If you asked the average person on the street where they get

When you adopt a plant-based lifestyle, you are consuming naturally occurring carbohydrates that feed your cells and breathe health and well-being into your body. You don't need to be afraid of carbohydrates; in fact, you need to embrace them as your best friend. Incorporate them into every meal. Your brain, cells, organs, vessels, and body will love you for it.

their protein, they will say it is in the meat that they eat. Moreover, they honestly believe that meat is the only protein source.

Cutting Out the MiddleMan

What is ironic about people's belief about protein and meat is that protein actually originates in plants, not animals. These are the people who don't want anything to do with plants on their plate. Plants are the original protein source. The way protein gets into a steak, lamb chop, chicken leg, or pork roast happens when the animal is alive and consumes protein in plants (grass, oats, wheat, soy). The protein is then transferred into the flesh of the animal. When you eat meat, you are consuming a secondary source of protein. The added "perk" when you eat meat is that it comes in a nice cholesterol-, hormone-, and fat-laden package.

If you can get all of the protein you need by eating whole, plant-based foods, you do not need to eat meat and put your health at risk. Plants are the source of all our nutritional needs. This may be something you were never aware of and are just learning for the first time. It may be overwhelming for you to absorb this right now. That is okay. If you have heard this before that is okay too. Sometimes we need to hear something many times before it rings that bell. By the end of this book, you will feel more confident in this knowledge through the resources, references, and

Consumption of large amounts of animal protein has been shown to negatively affect health.

information shared, and then hopefully you will do your own research to further support the information you have been provided. Remember—this is a journey, your journey.

How much protein should you be consuming each day? For women, the average amount of protein needed is about 46 grams and for men, it is about 56 grams. [14] These values are approximate and may vary a bit depending on your age, whether you are immunocompromised, your athletic activity, and if you are pregnant. In reality, the average American consumes much more than is ever needed and most of the protein consumed is animal-based. Researchers have shown that you can have too much of a good thing with protein, especially if the source is from animals. Consumption of large amounts of animal protein has been shown to negatively affect health. [16] A connection exists

We get our daily calories from three main groups: fats, carbohydrates, and proteins.

between the amount of animal protein consumed and death from cardiovascular disease. In contrast, people who had a high plant protein intake had

The Three Amigos

Put simply, we get our daily calories from three main groups of nutrients: fats, carbohydrates,

less mortality from cardiovascular disease, cancer, and other causes. [17] The source of your protein is of utmost concern. It has been demonstrated in scientific studies that we may process plant protein differently than animal protein, so more is okay as long as it is plant-based protein. [15] If you focus on plants for your protein, you will reduce your risk of disease and death from cardiovascular disease, cancer, and other lifestyle-related diseases. When someone asks you, and they will, where you get your protein, you can say from plants—the same place where elephants, rhinos, hippos, and gorillas get their protein.

and proteins. We need all three. All for one and one for all. By limiting one or more groups, you automatically shift your calorie intake to another, upsetting our body's natural function and causing deficiencies and a host of other metabolic issues. We need to honor the way our bodies are meant to function and not starve our systems from the very nutrients they require.

One thing is true however: the source and quality of the fats, carbs, and proteins that we consume determines our health and well-being. We want our fats, carbs, and proteins from whole, plant-based foods.

Whole Plant-Based Foods

What are whole, plant-based foods? They are foods that are derived from plants as close to their natural form with minimal processing. They include all vegetables, fruits, whole grains, legumes, nuts, and seeds in their pure form or slightly processed, such as oats, flours, flavorings, and spices. The further the food is from its original form, the more processed it is and the less nutritional value it contains. For instance, a wheat berry (the

origin of wheat flour) is wheat in its purest form, but as it is dried, milled, and ground into flour, it becomes more and more processed and loses more of its nutritional value. Eating corn on the cob is consuming corn in its purest form. As it is dried, milled, and ground into corn flour it becomes more and more processed. Olive oil is basically removing the natural olive from the equation and consuming only its expressed oils.

Why Should We Eat Healthily?

Living an excellent life so that we are not crippled and riddled with sickness and pain now and in our later years is the reason we should eat healthily. If you have ever suffered from a debilitating illness such as heart disease, cancer, dementia, or rheumatoid arthritis, or had the terrible experience of watching a parent, friend or relative suffer, then you understand the urgency of finding a way to prevent these diseases from occurring. As we will see later, our diets (good or bad) play a major role in determining our health and well-being.

Why Should You Eat Vegetables?

Vegetables are naturally low in calories and provide nutrients vital for health—they are nutrient-dense. People who consume more vegetables in their daily diet are more likely to have a reduced risk of many chronic diseases such as heart disease, hypertension, cancer, autoimmune disease, and diabetes. [18] A diet rich in vegetables, of all types and colors, will provide a full spectrum of nutrients and vitamins, including micronutrients and macronutrients, essential amino acids, proteins, minerals, complex carbohydrates, and fiber.

Eating vegetables does not mean that you only munch on some lettuce leaves or crunch on some carrot sticks. There are

People who consume more vegetables in their daily diet are more likely to have a reduced risk of many chronic diseases.

countless ways to prepare an abundance of vegetable varieties, so much so that you can eat a different vegetable prepared in a different way for an entire year and never get bored. In this book, you will learn how to prepare your food in a tasty and exciting way.

Are Fruits Good for You?

The answer to this is a resounding YES! Besides their wonderful sweetness and deliciousness, fruits are packed with a multitude of nutrients, vitamins, minerals, proteins, and fiber. It seems like every day we hear from the media about some new research study that proclaims the benefits of consuming this or that fruit. From their cholesterol-lowering, heart-healing, and cancer- and disease-fighting properties, fruits, along with their vegetable brethren, are the superheroes of the natural food world.

The ability of fruit to negatively affect blood sugar levels is a misnomer. Consumption of whole fruit in its natural form actually has a balancing effect on blood glucose levels. While all carbohydrates will affect blood sugar to some degree, it is the package it comes in that will determine how much.

Current State of Eating & Health

As a society, the way we eat on a daily basis is centered on fast and tasty. The Standard American Diet is, unfortunately, becoming the Standard (insert your country here) Diet. We have become a fast-food-, processed-food-world, and, as a result, the incidence of lifestyle diseases is skyrocketing around the globe.

On US soil, over half of Americans have heart disease, 1.8 million are diagnosed with cancer each year, 34 million have diabetes, and 89 million have pre-diabetes. In addition to those diagnosed, heart disease and cancer are the top killers with over 1.2 million Americans dying from these diseases each year. Worldwide, over 18 million suffer from cancer with 9.5 million dying from it annually. Heart disease is the number one killer worldwide, accounting for over 17.9 million deaths each year. Diabetes has a stunning worldwide incidence of 422 million. Obesity wins the prize, with rates at an all-time high and a worldwide projection of 3.28 billion diagnosed as overweight or obese by 2030. [19] [20] [21] [22] [23] [24] [25]

These are all unacceptable statistics, and they do not bode well for our future. Fortunately for all of us, the answer to avoiding unnecessary disease and death lies within our control and at the end of our fork.

Chapter 3

WHAT YOU DON'T NEED

•••

NO NAPs!

No, this plan is not about never taking a nap—this plan is about No Oils, No Animal Products (NO NAPs). This probably sounds extreme to most people, but once you realize the benefits of eating whole, plant-based foods and the wealth of options and choices available, you will never look at this way of eating as restrictive.

Why do the WFPB20 Lifestyle Plan?

In order to be successful on this plan, you will want to believe in the **"why"** you are doing this. This is important especially if this way of eating is very new to you. You have to feel comfortable and believe in what you are doing. You have to be able to walk-the-walk and talk-the-talk.

Without a doubt, when you adopt a plant-based lifestyle, you will get lots of questions and comments from others who may or may not agree with what you are doing. They will be concerned about your protein consumption, almost to obsession. For some people, the foods you eat threaten the foods they eat, especially if they are not eating healthy. This may bring up feelings of guilt, fear, anger, or resentment in others. Remember, these are their feelings and not yours. You do not have

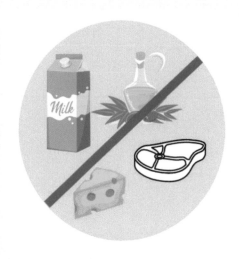

responsibility for the feelings of others. You need to take care of yourself and let them take care of themselves. If they ask, you may share what you are doing and why. Sometimes all is needed to allay their fears is to understand the why. However, only offer an explanation when directly asked and keep it short. Continue the conversation organically if they express more interest.

Why No Meat?

So, let's explore the reasons behind the replacement of calorie-dense meat (beef, pork, lamb, poultry, wild game, and fish) in our diets with nutrient-dense vegetables, fruits, whole grains, beans, legumes, nuts, and seeds, and why this will lead

CHOLESTEROL (MG) CONTENT
(3.5 oz serving size)

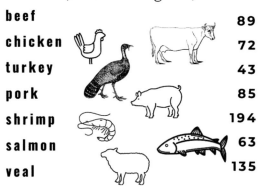

beef	89
chicken	72
turkey	43
pork	85
shrimp	194
salmon	63
veal	135

> "People eat meat thinking they will become strong as an ox, forgetting that the ox eats grass" ~ Pino Caruso

to improved health, weight loss, and overall wellness.

Remember, even if you are eating grass-fed, free-range, antibiotic-free, no-added hormones meat, you are still consuming all of the hormones, toxins, and chemicals that an animal has naturally running through its blood. Those substances are not natural to humans and have a definite impact on human health when consumed. Here are 20 reasons why you should consider avoiding meat in your meals.

20 REASONS To Not Eat Meat

1. Meat contains protein, but along with that protein you get **fat, cholesterol, antibiotics, hormones, additives, toxins**, no fiber, and few nutrients.
2. Meat is a calorie-dense food and plant-based whole foods are nutrient-dense foods.
3. Meat does not contain fiber. All plants contain fiber.

4. Meat does not make you strong. Meat consumption leads to inflammation and disease.
5. Meat has been directly linked to colon cancer. [1] [2]
6. Processed meat has been classified as a Group I known carcinogen. [3]
7. Meat consumption has been linked to inflammation. [4]
8. Meat consumption has been linked to heart disease. [5][6][7]
9. Meat consumption has been directly linked to breast cancer. [8][9]
10. Meat consumption has been linked to kidney cancer. [10]
11. All meat contains artery-damaging cholesterol, including beef, chicken, pork, turkey, fish, and shellfish.
12. All meat contains disease-causing saturated fats.
13. Meat contains animal hormones which are treated as invaders in the human body.
14. People who eat meat have decreased longevity. [11]
15. Meat consumption is linked to impotence in men. [12]
16. Meat consumption may have an adverse effect on fertility. [13]
17. Eating meat is correlated with obesity. [14]
18. Athletic performance can be impaired from inflammation due to meat consumption. [15]
19. Meat consumption may be related to a moderate increase in depression. [16]
20. Eating red meat can fast forward the body's biological clock. [17]

Why You Don't Need Dairy or Eggs

It may be overwhelming to entertain the possibility of eliminating dairy. Many of us have been consuming dairy in one form or another for most of our lives. Studies abound discussing the harmful effects of dairy and eggs including heart disease, cancer, diabetes, infant apnea, inflammation, autoimmune disorders, high blood pressure, and high cholesterol, among others. If the thought of leaving behind all of your beloved meats, cheeses, creamers, and eggs frightens and stresses you, please be comforted. Today, there are a plethora of meat-free and dairy-free alternatives for these products including burgers, sausages, ground beef, chicken, fish, milks, creamers, whipped cream, yogurts, sour cream, cream cheese, hard cheeses, cheese slices, mozzarella, and Parmesan-like cheeses. The choices are vast. The same can be said for eggs, where

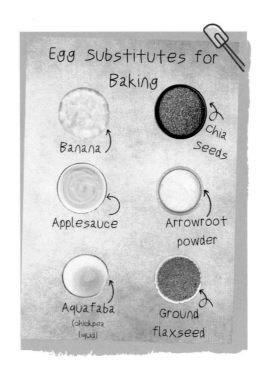

Egg Substitutes for Baking

Banana

Chia seeds

Applesauce

Arrowroot powder

Aquafaba (chickpea liquid)

Ground flaxseed

new products are popping up in stores at a rapid pace. Some egg substitutes are available for baking and some that cook up like real eggs. This makes the transition to a meat-, dairy-, and egg-free diet so much easier, not to mention healthier. Take it as slow or as fast as you need— using the meat and dairy-free

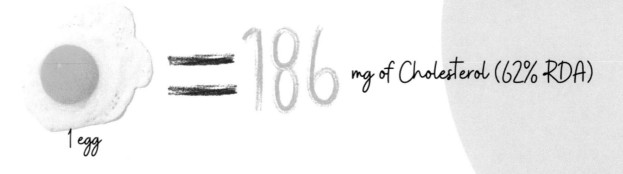

1 egg = 186 mg of Cholesterol (62% RDA)

substitutes as a lifeline to better health, happiness, and wellness.

Explore the options and see what fits for you. A significant percentage of these substitutes are processed foods and contain unhealthy ingredients but at the very least do not contain animal products. Each person will be different as they travel this journey. Some of you will be able to kick meat, dairy and eggs to the curb and never look back, others will have a more circuitous route to a meat-, dairy- and egg-free diet.

Remember, you have to do what works for you, otherwise you will not be successful. The goal is for you to be successful as you travel to better wellness.

Next, let's explore the reasons behind the replacement of calorie-dense dairy (milk, cheese, and derivatives) and eggs in our diets with nutrient-dense vegetables, fruits, whole grains, beans, legumes, nuts, and seeds, and why this will lead to improved health, weight loss, and overall wellness. Here are 20 compelling reasons.

 ## REASONS To Not Eat Dairy or Eggs

1. Milk products increase the risk of cancer. [18] [19]
2. Dairy and egg products do not contain fiber.
3. Cow's milk is designed to grow a 65 lb newborn calf to a 700+ lb animal in less than one year. Imagine what it does for a child?
4. Milk does NOT do a body good. [20]
5. Cow's milk frequently contains antibiotics, insulin growth factor (IGF-1), estrogen, and synthetic hormones.
6. Cholesterol in dairy and in eggs has been linked to heart disease. [21]
7. The consumption of dairy products in infancy is linked to Type I diabetes. [22]

8. Milk protein can increase the production of IGF-1. [23]

9. Milk lactose can increase levels of inflammation. [24]

10. Drinking milk can expose one to the estrogen and progesterone of lactating cows.

11. There is a strong association between the consumption of dairy and prostate cancer. [25] [26]

12. Dairy and eggs have been linked to triple-negative breast cancer. [27]

13. Dairy has been found to have acne-promoting effects. [28]

14. Dairy has been found to trigger histamine responses in some individuals. [29]

15. Eliminating dairy products has been found to have a positive outcome for patients with schizophrenia. [30]

16. Dairy contains casomorphins shown to have addictive properties. [31]

17. Just one half of an egg per day has been associated with a higher risk of death. [32]

18. Milk-free diets have been associated with a decrease in cerebral folate deficiency in children. [33]

19. Consumption of dairy has indicated a positive association with Parkinson's Disease, especially in men. [34]

20. A positive association was found between milk and acne and other skin conditions. [35]

Why No Oil?

The oil on your lips is the fat on your hips. This is actually true for all oils. They are 100% fat. Although some oils contain a very small amount of micronutrients, the fat calories far outweigh the benefit you would gain. It makes much more sense to eat a cup of broccoli and get more nutritional benefit and not the empty fat calories you get from oil. Plus, broccoli is much more filling than a couple of tablespoons of oil. Why is this? Oil is devoid of fiber, whereas broccoli is loaded with fiber.

What about coconut oil and olive oil? There has been much written about how coconut oil and olive oil have many health benefits. These oils are great on the outside of our bodies like on our skin. However, they wreak havoc on the inside of our bodies. The only benefit one may be seeing is that these oils are typically eaten with veggies and that those benefits are masking the negative benefits of the oil. In actuality, the body is

working hard to strip some of the vital nutrients from the vegetables from under the mountain of pure fat. The benefits are coming from the whole food, not processed fat.

To be clear, not all oils are bad. There are natural oils in whole foods such as avocados, nuts, seeds, and really all plant-based sources. Some have a lot of oil in them and some have limited. When the oil is packaged inside fiber- and nutrition-filled packages, then that's the kind of oil you want to consume.

Don't worry about the cooking issue with oils. This book will show you how to cook without oil! Yes, you read it correctly. No-oil cooking. It is really easy, and your heart and endothelial cells will love you for it.

The Significance of Processed Foods

Processed food is any food that does not look like it did when it first came from the soil. For example, an apple that you purchase in a store

looks like it did when it was picked from the tree. Tomatoes, potatoes, bananas, watermelon, and pineapple are additional examples.

When you purchase wheat flour, wheat pasta, or wheat bread, it does not resemble the long, golden-shafted plant grown in fields throughout the world. These are processed foods. Meaning that they have undergone a transformation from the way they looked when they were harvested from the soil.

There are degrees of processing. Many kinds of pasta, flour, and bread can be classified as minimally processed. The wheat that they are made from was harvested and then ground down to flour. Depending on how much grinding was done, you can have the less minimally processed whole wheat flour or the more processed white flour. From there, the flours can be used in combination with other processes and ingredients to make doughs, pasta, and many other products. The more transformations they go through, and the more ingredients are added, the more processed the food becomes. Pineapple is unprocessed whereas cream-filled and iced pineapple cupcakes are very processed.

The further you get from the original form, the less nutrient-dense the food gets. Food manufacturers may remove nutrients such as the healthier part of the grain, so the product has a longer shelf-life. Or they may add ingredients to make the product more appealing to the general public such as oils, fats, additives, salt, flavorings, colorings, preservatives, thickeners, stabilizers, pesticides, toxins, and emulsifiers, to name a

WHOLE FOOD VS OIL

	Olives	100 gms	Olive Oil
calories	115		884
fat	11.3g		100g
fiber	3.2g		0
carbs	5.4g		0
protein	0.9g		0

	Coconut*		Coconut Oil*
calories	160		388
fat	15g		45
fiber	4g		0
carbs	6.8g		0
protein	1.5g		0

*values are based on 45g of coconut vs oil

few. There is a whole industry dedicated to creating processed foods that stimulate our natural senses and desires for salty, sugary, fatty foods. They trigger cravings and lead to addictions, overeating, and disease.

Organic versus Non-Organic

What is the difference between organic and non-organic plant-based foods? Do health and nutritional benefits exist for one over the other? In the US, the labeling of foods as organic is strictly regulated by the US Department of Agriculture (USDA). Basically speaking, 100% certified organic applies to single-ingredient foods (some multi-ingredient foods if each item is certified organic) that follow rigorous procedures for the growing and harvesting of crops. This includes soil that has not been contaminated with chemicals over the past three years, no use of synthetic fertilizers or pesticides, no irradiation or genetic engineering practices, and no introduction of antibiotics or growth hormones. Organic farmers can use predatory insects, mulch, crop rotation, green and livestock manure, and on rare last resort occasions, and only if in conjunction with USDA consultants, use a few permitted natural and synthetic pesticides. These foods will be labeled with the USDA organic seal.

These guidelines should help you when you are shopping and looking for organic labeling. Single-ingredient foods should have 100% certified organic on their labels. More processed foods will indicate if some or all of their ingredients are organic. Read the labels carefully to ensure you are buying what you want. The Environmental Working Group produces an annual list that includes the Clean 15 and Dirty Dozen produce guide that you can use when shopping.

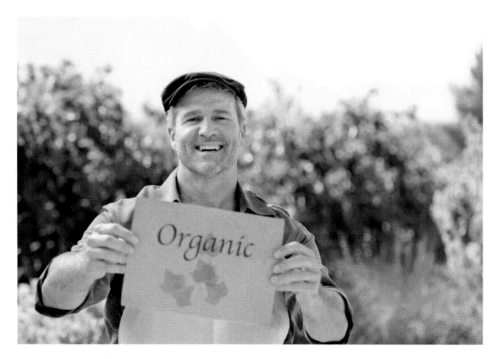

Organic produce typically has lower detectable levels of pesticides and has been found to have higher levels of some nutrients. Organic produce typically cost more than non-organic produce due to stricter farming practices however, it may not be necessary to buy all organic produce. And while eating organic produce is better in some cases than non-organic, this should be a secondary consideration. The most important is that eating any fruit or vegetable is far better than eating meat, dairy, or processed foods

Clean 15 vs. Dirty Dozen*

1. cauliflower	1. strawberries
2. broccoli	2. nectarines
3. avocado	3. cherries
4. cantaloupe	4. celery
5. sweet corn	5. tomatoes
6. mushrooms	6. potatoes
7. pineapple	7. apples
8. honeydew	8. grapes
9. onions	9. peaches
10. cabbage	10. pears
11. kiwi	11. kale
12. papaya	12. raisins
13. sweet peas	
14. asparagus	
15. eggplant	

*Environmental Working Group 2020. Raisins tested for the first time but not yet officially added to the list

Chapter Four

FIBER IS YOUR FRIEND

Fiber & Constipation

An estimated 15-20% of the population, or more than 50 million people, suffers from chronic constipation, spending billions of dollars on laxatives and medical treatments. [1] This does not include those who do not go to the doctor for their constipation issues and treat themselves with over-the-counter medicines.

In 2016, Americans spent over $1.3 billion dollars on over-the-counter laxatives. It is the most frequent illness seen by gastro-enterologists and takes up at least 50% of their patient care time. [2] Why are so many people suffering from constipation? Could it have something to do with the way we eat? The foods we put into our body? You can avoid most constipation issues simply by including fiber in your diet. The recommended fiber intake is around 35-40 grams of fiber per day, yet Americans get less than 15 grams per day. [3] No wonder we are a constipated group of people.

What is the Importance of Fiber?

We have all seen the commercials on TV: a cereal, snack, or processed food contains this mysterious ingredient called fiber and if you buy this product your life will be wonderful. Or a very trustworthy-looking person complains of their constipation and tells us that simply taking this fiber supplement every day solves all of their problems and we see them dance happily across the TV screen. The messaging regarding fiber is often confusing and therefore, it is important to understand the science.

Fiber is the dietary material or bulk-containing substance only found in plant-based foods, which is resistant to the action of digestive enzymes. It is really that simple. Think of the texure of an apple, orange, or celery.

Sponge & Plunger

Fiber comes in both soluble and insoluble forms. Soluble fiber simply means it actually dissolves in water. Examples of foods containing soluble fiber are oats, peas, beans, apples, citrus fruits, and carrots. Soluble fiber absorbs water and changes its form to a more gelatinous nature. Our gut bacteria go to work on it as it passes through the digestive system.

Insoluble fiber, like its name, does not dissolve in water and does not change its form. It looks the same as it does going in as it does going out. Our gut bacteria work on insoluble fiber as well. If your gut bacteria are not used to seeing fiber come through, there will be an adjustment period while fiber-digesting bacteria replace the non-fiber digesting bacteria. Each form of fiber, soluble and insoluble, has a job to do. This is where the sponge and the plunger analogy comes in. Soluble fiber, serving as a sponge, soaks up all of the bad stuff in our system like toxins, drugs, chemicals, cholesterol, hormones, and waste products. The insoluble fiber, pushing along unwanted substances and acting like a plunger, comes from behind plunging it all out of our bodies as waste. A perfect team!

Take a look at the top 20 benefits of eating fiber. By including more fiber in your diet you will have less desire to add unhealthy foods to your body. You will want to focus on whole, plant-based foods that naturally contain fiber and stay away from processed foods with added fiber. Remember, nutrient-dense, not calorie-dense, is the key to weight control and true health. With WFPB20, you will get plenty of both soluble and insoluble fiber and your gut, heart, and body will thank you for it.

 REASONS Why You Should Love Fiber

1. Fiber helps eliminate harmful substances from our bodies by soaking them up and moving them out of circulation.
2. Fiber helps keep us feeling satiated after meals and triggers the brain's satiation mechanism.

3. Fiber is the key to weight loss and weight control by filling you up and making you less likely to binge eat. [4]
4. Fiber helps to stabilize our blood sugar by slowing down the release of sugars to the bloodstream.
5. Fiber reduces the risk of prostate cancer. [5]
6. Fiber helps to prevent heart disease by helping to remove inflammatory products. [6]
7. Fiber helps to prevent diabetes by slowing the absorption of sugar and steadying blood sugar levels. [7]
8. Fiber helps to prevent colon cancer. A diet high in fiber lowers your risk of colon cancer by keeping your bowels moving regularly and eliminating toxins. [8] [9]
9. Fiber helps to alleviate menopause symptoms. [10]
10. Fiber helps reduce the risk of breast cancer. [10]
11. Fiber reduces the risk of mouth and throat cancers. [11]
12. Insoluble fiber helps prevent diverticulosis, a condition that causes small pockets to form throughout your intestinal tract. [12]
13. Fiber helps to reduce cholesterol levels in the blood.
14. Fiber helps to improve digestive health by softening and adding bulk to the stool.
15. Fiber helps to rid the body of excess harmful estrogen.
16. Fiber helps with the side effects of chemotherapy by helping to expel the drugs from the body.
17. Fiber helps reduce inflammation associated with arthritis. [13]
18. Fiber helps to boost the body's immune system. [14]
19. Fiber helps to build a healthy gut biome. [14]
20. Fiber has been shown to extend longevity. [15]

Chapter Five

EAT YOUR BEANS & GREENS AT EVERY MEAL

• •

Beans (Legumes)

Across the globe, people who included legumes as part of their daily diet have been found to be among the healthiest and live the longest. [1] From black beans to chickpeas to cannellini, kidney, or pinto, beans and other legumes (like lentils, edamame, and split peas) provide an easy and affordable way to get many of the critical nutrients you need to thrive.

Whether you use canned, frozen, fresh, or dried, you are getting a healthy dose of nutrients and fiber. A serving of 1 cup of beans can provide over 15 grams of protein, 28 grams of carbohydrates, 5 grams of fiber, and just 2 grams of fat, which represents a fairly significant portion of our daily require- ments. They are an excellent food especially for heart health, diabetes control, cancer preven- tion, weight loss, seniors, and athletes. [2] [3] [4]

Beans are versatile ingredi- ents in many recipes. They can be used in soups, stews, chilis, sauces, salads, pasta, casse- roles, dips, and spreads and are featured in most ethnic foods. Try including them in some form or another for most of your meals.

Greens

Leafy green vegetables should be a part of every healthy diet. They are filled with vitamins, minerals, phytonutrients, and fiber. Study after study has shown that eating leafy greens can help lower the risk of heart disease, obesity, diabetes, cancer, and physical and mental decline. [5] [6] [7] [8] [9]

What Kind of Leafy Greens Should You Eat?

Leafy greens come in all shapes and sizes. Included in

this list are kale, swiss chard, bok choy, broccoli, spinach, collard greens, and Brussels sprouts. In adopting WFPB20, the important thing is to include a variety of greens in your diet. Each type of leafy green brings its own unique value to your meal. They provide excellent nutrition, and comple- ment and enhance the benefits of one another. You should aim for 3-5 servings of leafy greens each and every day to ensure the best of health. If you have been diagnosed with heart disease,

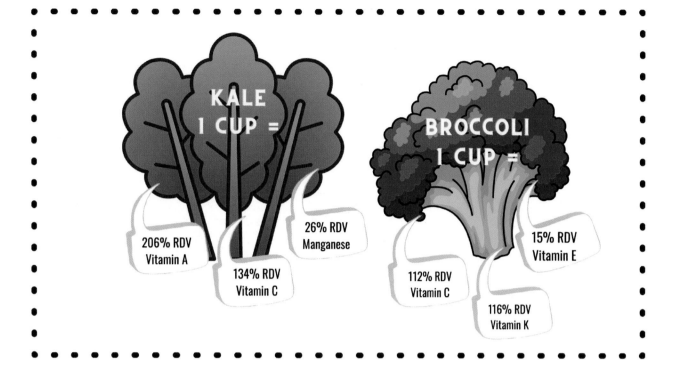

Dr. Caldwell Esselstyn recommends that you eat 6 servings (handfuls) of steamed greens topped with a little balsamic vinegar every day to keep your blood vessels healthy. [10]

Why is Chewing Your Greens Important?

A chain reaction occurs when we chew our greens. The chewing action stimulates enzymes in our saliva where they aid in converting the nitrates found in greens to nitrite. Maximizing the amount of nitrites produced is important because they go on to be converted into nitric oxide in the gut tract. The nitric oxide is crucial for the endothelial cells that line all of our blood vessels in staying healthy and flexible. This in turn helps to reduce the risk of cardiovascular disease and a host of other ailments from occurring.

WHY WE CHEW OUR GREENS

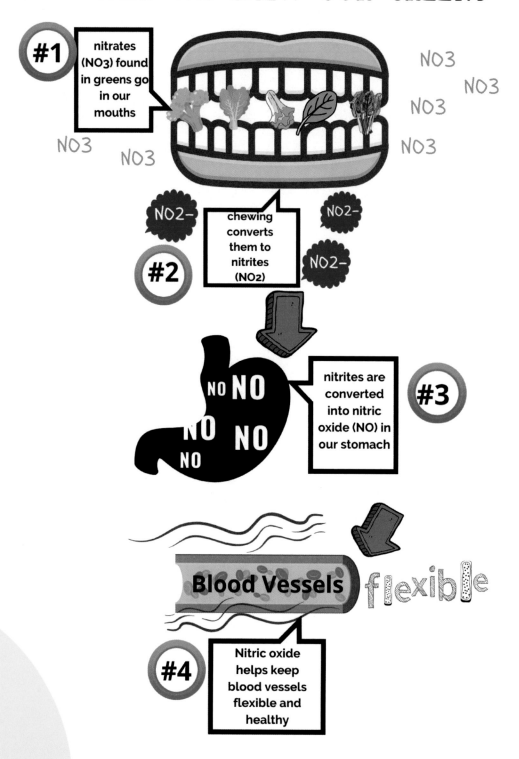

#1 nitrates (NO3) found in greens go in our mouths

NO3 NO3 NO3 NO3 NO3 NO3 NO3

#2 chewing converts them to nitrites (NO2)

NO2− NO2− NO2−

#3 nitrites are converted into nitric oxide (NO) in our stomach

NO NO NO NO NO

Blood Vessels flexible

#4 Nitric oxide helps keep blood vessels flexible and healthy

Chapter Six

RISK OF LIFESTYLE DISEASES

· ·

What is a Lifestyle Disease?

Lifestyle diseases are caused primarily through our daily actions, like eating, drinking, and physical activity. For most people, diet has a greater effect on health than any other factor.

As we read previously, the standard diets worldwide are increasingly filled with fat, sugar, salt, meat, dairy, oil, processed and fast foods, and very little vegetables, fruits, and whole grains.

Common sense prevails in the thinking that if we continue on this route, bad things are going to happen to our health. Obesity, cardiovascular diseases, diabetes, autoimmune disease, infertility, rheumatoid arthritis, and neurodegenerative disorders are all examples of lifestyle diseases that affect more and more people each year.

Obesity

Being overweight and obese are lifestyle disorders defined as abnormal or excessive fat accumulation that may result in adverse health effects. The prevalence of obesity has rapidly increased over the past 20 years becoming a national and global epidemic with over 1.9 billion adults and 340 million children classified as being overweight or obese. [1] Medical costs for health effects due to being overweight or obese in the US alone range from $147 to $210 billion. [2]

Excessive fat cells produce hormones that can override the body's normal function and unbalance a person's health and well-being. As we have seen, fiber-containing foods can aid in weight loss and increased health. The road to better health and weight loss is through a whole-food, plant-based lifestyle.

Cardiovascular Disease

Cardiovascular disease (CVD) is the leading cause of death worldwide, causing over 17.9 million deaths annually—with America and Germany ranking first and second, respectively. [3] Cardiovascular disease is actually a collection of disorders affecting the heart and its blood vessels and includes coronary heart disease and stroke. Clogging of the arteries is the leading cause of CVD which is related to lifestyle including diet and physical activity. Artery-clogging foods (cholesterol and fat-laden) are the main culprit.

The Importance of Our Endothelium

Endothelial cells make up the endothelium, the single-celled-thick inner lining of all of our blood vessels. They play a crucial role in wound healing, controlling inflammation, serve as the brain-blood barrier, are implicated in diabetes, cardiovascular disease, and a host of other diseases and conditions. When healthy, they can repel substances from adhering to blood vessel walls, prevent blood clots, help the flow of blood, and produce nitric oxide, which keeps the vessels flexible and strong. They actually control the widening and narrowing of our blood vessels, which controls the amount of blood flow at any giving time. Depending on their location, they serve different functions. They are selectively permeable meaning that they allow some substances through to the surrounding cells and tissues and keep out others. They work both ways in that they also control the movement of substances from our cells and tissue into our bloodstream. Damage to their function is tied to diabetes, pulmonary disease, inflammatory disease, cardiovascular disease, strokes, neurological disorders, and immune disorders. [4] Endothelium cells promote tissue growth and repair. They are also crucial in the formation of new blood vessels which has implications for cancer and its spread throughout the body.

Damage occurs to our vessels by way of chemicals and toxins that travel through our blood system. Saturated fats, elevated blood sugar, sodium, triglycerides, cholesterol, hormones, pesticides, smoking, alcohol, and drugs are among the substances that can do substantial damage. Oxidizing substances wreak havoc on the lining of the blood vessels causing an inflammatory response. Over time, with continual exposure to these substances, the health of the endothelium degrades as well as the health of our bodies. Foods that can help heal and prevent vessel damage contain omega-3 fatty acids, antioxidants, vitamins B6 and B12, folic acid, and fiber, once again indicating that diet changes can substantially reduce the incidence of heart disease.

Cancer

While all cancers are not lifestyle-related, a substantial number of them are related to our diets. At the very least, prevention and or recovery can happen when we pay attention to what we feed our bodies. With over 18 million diagnosed with cancer worldwide and 9.5 million deaths per year, it's time we pay attention to causes and not just treat the symptoms. [5] [6] Studies abound related to our diets and the incidence of cancer. We know from the science that has been presented so far that the consumption of animal products is correlated to many different types of cancer. Conversely, eating a whole-food, plant-based diet, full of antioxidants and anti-cancer fighting nutrients, has been shown to challenge cancer cells from ever taking hold in our bodies.

Diabetes

More than 34 million Americans have diabetes and approximately 31 million of these have type II diabetes. [7] Over 1.6 million die from diabetes complications each year. Worldwide, cases soar beyond 460 million. [8] There are two main types of diabetes: type I and type II. Type I diabetics are unable to produce insulin and this is usually genetic and evident fairly early in life. Type II diabetics do not produce enough insulin. This disease is, for the most part, related directly to the foods we put into our bodies. Elevated blood sugar and an overabundance of fats lead to a dysfunction in insulin production.

What is Blood Sugar?

Blood sugar, or glucose, is the main sugar that flows through our blood broken down from the different foods we eat. Glucose provides our body with the energy it needs in order to function. This is why it is very important to have enough glucose in our blood.

Glucose is King.

In fact, it is both king and queen of the body. Without glucose, most of us would eventually die. It is the primary food the brain needs to live as well as every living cell in our body. Can the body survive without glucose and just live on ketones or fat? For a length of time, sure, but there is much controversy regarding whether this is healthy in the long term for our bodies. Our bodies prefer glucose because it is easier to convert into the energy we need. When we eat starchy foods, glucose from the breakdown of these foods travels through our blood system. The rate at which these foods breakdown is a function of the quality of the food. If we are consuming whole, plant-based foods then

GLYCEMIC FOODS INDEX

The glycemic index, or GI, is a measure of how a carbohydrate-containing food raises blood glucose. The rise and fall of our blood glucose levels greatly affect our physical being.

LOW GLYCEMIC INDEX (55 OR LOWER)		MEDIUM GLYCEMIC INDEX (56 THROUGH 69)		HIGH GLYCEMIC INDEX (70+)
Apples	Hazelnuts	Banana	Brown Rice	Watermelon
Oranges	Corn Tortillas	Pineapple	Honey	Winter Squash
Blueberries	Whole Grain Pasta	Kiwi	Cashews	Frozen Corn
Strawberries	Spaghetti	Beets	Macadamia	White Wheat
Raspberries	Soy Milk	Carrots		White Rice
Peaches	Olives	Corn on Cob		Potato
Plums		Sweet Potato		Rice Crackers
Cherries		Plantain		Dried Dates
Chickpeas		Pinto Beans		Pretzels
Lentils		Kidney Beans		Chips
Soy Beans		Green Peas		Candy
Almonds		Rolled Oats		Processed Cereals
Peanuts		Pita		White Sugar
Walnuts		Cornmeal		White Flours
Pecans		Popcorn		Most Breads
Sunflower Seeds		Whole Grain Bread		
		Udon Noodles		

Source: [19]

the breakdown will be a slow, steady process. This is because those foods contain fiber, micro and macronutrients, and complex carbohydrates and sugars. If we are consuming processed carbohydrates, then the breakdown is rapid. Blood sugar spikes quickly and then, just as quickly, it falls, leaving us lethargic and listless.

In a normally functioning body, these glucose molecules need to get into the cells so it can provide fuel for the cell. It does this through insulin.

What is Insulin?

Insulin, which is a hormone and produced by the pancreas, is the conduit to getting glucose into the cells. The body has an amazing ability to detect glucose in the body and to instantly ramp up its insulin production to match the amount of glucose present.

How does insulin do its job? Think of insulin like a lock to a key—the key to the "door" of a cell. The insulin picks up each glucose molecule and transports it to the muscle or fat cells. The cell surface recognizes the insulin "key" and unlocks the entry allowing for the admission of the glucose molecule.

What is Insulin Resistance?

Insulin resistance occurs when the mechanism for recognizing or accepting insulin by the cells fails. This happens most frequently when there is too much fat in the cells blocking the entryway for glucose to enter. Insulin then builds up in the bloodstream along with the glucose. The pancreas becomes fatigued at continuing

to produce insulin, and the system crashes.

What is a Type II Diabetes Diagnosis?

Type II diabetes is recognized as a body's inability to effectively regulate glucose levels in the bloodstream. Most people with diabetes have type II diabetes. They also most likely suffer from excess body weight and have low levels of physical activity. They have higher levels of fat in and around their organs and muscle which interferes in the transport of glucose into cells. Unstable blood sugar levels, frequent urination, extreme thirst, constant hunger, and fatigue can all be symptoms.

Can Type II Diabetes be Prevented or Reversed?

There is a plethora of science out there showing that people who change their diets to one that is whole-food, plant-based, can not only prevent but can also reverse type II diabetes. Simply by removing processed foods and adding more fruits, vegetables and fiber to their plates can result in a gradual reduction and/or elimination of the need for insulin medication.

Autoimmune Diseases

The classification of autoimmune diseases includes diseases where our immune systems attack our own body's tissues. There are over 100 of these chronic debilitating diseases including Crohn's, multiple sclerosis, lupus, rheumatoid arthritis, psoriasis, celiac, Hashimoto's, ulcerative colitis, type I diabetes, and scleroderma. These diseases have skyrocketed in numbers over the past years where now over 4% of people worldwide suffer from one or more of these diseases. [9] The role of diets containing high fat, cholesterol, protein, sugar, and sodium and high consumption of fast food and processed foods have been shown to be instigators in the occurrence of autoimmune diseases. [10] This indicates once again how the control of whether we are diagnosed with these diseases is at the end of our forks.

Infertility

Although some infertility issues can stem from genetic factors, many fertility issues can be addressed with proper nutrition. Obesity is known to disrupt normal hormone cycles in the body which in turn affect the reproductive organs in a woman's body. Toxins and animal hormones in the food we eat can also impact our own hormone cycles. Clearing your diet of these dangerous substances can prevent and even reverse fertility issues. Enhancing your health with whole, plant-based foods can encourage healthy hormonal function.

Dementia and Alzheimer's

Worldwide, over 50 million people suffer from some form of dementia. Alzheimer's, which is a form of dementia, makes up about 60-70% of that. [11] Despite the common nature of dementia in the elderly and sometimes in younger patients, this is not believed to be a natural progression of age. Dementia including Alzheimer's disease has not been found to be reversible, however, there may be ways to prevent it from occurring in the first place.

Researchers have found a link between Alzheimer's and plaque and cholesterol accumulation in the blood vessels that feed the brain. Low blood flow to the brain as a result of these blockages increases the risk of dementia including Alzheimer's. Studies have shown that diets rich in sugars, fats, and processed foods have been linked to a decline in cognitive function and an increase in the risk of Alzheimer's. Foods high in antioxidants, vitamin A, folate, and iron are all indicated in being helpful in fighting cognitive impairment. In the Harvard Women's Health Study, a diet high in fat content showed a significant impact on cognition whereas consuming fruits, specifically berries and vegetable juices, were correlated with improved cognitive function. [12]

Osteoporosis & Bone Health

Osteoporosis is a disease that is manifested by low bone density and deterioration of the actual bone structure, resulting in low bone strength. A fracture resulting from osteoporosis happens every 3 seconds, worldwide. [13] For people over the age of 50, the rate of a fall resulting in a fracture over the remainder of their life is 1 in every 3 women and 1 in every 5 men. It is estimated that for people who suffer from a hip fracture 20% of them will die within 6 months of their injury. [14] Bone health is very important in the health and wellbeing of everyone.

Calcium, along with Vitamin D, is crucial to the development and maintenance of strong bones. There is considerable conflicting research and science relating to the cause of osteoporosis including the consumption of dairy, the lack of weight-bearing exercise, and a diet that includes an excess of animal protein. Some researchers have indicated that it may be our diet that is causing calcium to be depleted from our bones. High protein foods like dairy, eggs, and meat are acidic. Our bodies adjust to the acidic foods by releasing calcium from our bones to neutralize our systems and in turn, this results in bone loss, weakness, and fractures.

Populations studied around the world indicate a correlation between dairy consumption and fracture rates. In three independent US studies, women who consumed more calcium from dairy had twice to three times the bone loss and fracture rates than women who consumed no dairy or obtained their calcium from plant sources. [15] [16] [17]. Dr. Colin Campbell, one of the authors of *The China Study*, states that "the association between the intake of animal protein and fracture rates appears to be as strong as that between cigarette smoking and lung cancer." Adopting a whole-food, plant-based lifestyle together with daily weight-bearing exercise are positive indicators of healthy and strong bones.

So far, we have learned that the nutritional value of the food you put into your body will, in part, determine your overall health.

What are the actual components of food that make it healthy? Macronutrients, micronutrients, phytonutrients, vitamins, minerals, and antioxidants are all important to consider when adopting WFPB20. You want to ensure that you are maximizing your nutritional intake to provide your body with all it needs for optimal performance.

Chapter Seven

NUTRITION BASICS

· ·

What are Vitamins and Minerals?

Vitamins are groups of organic compounds that are essential to the body and are made by living organisms. When you are following WFPB20, consuming no animal products, you are getting the best source of vitamins available, without the detrimental health effects. Vitamins are either water or fat-soluble. Every vitamin plays a role in your body's production of enzymes and/or proteins. Other crucial functions include nerve function, eye and skin health, digestive health, cell metabolism, and immune system health. Not all vitamins are readily available through plants. If you adopt a whole-food, plant-based lifestyle, then you will need to obtain your vitamin B12 and D by consuming fortified foods or through supplements. Your body can also make vitamin D through sun exposure, but then you risk your body to the dangers of too much sun.

While some vitamins are made by the body, minerals come from the earth. They are taken up by plants and then are transferred into our bodies when we eat the plants. There are essential minerals that are required daily, and they may include calcium, phosphorus, magnesium, sodium, chloride, potassium, sulfur. Trace minerals that are required in very small amounts include iron, manganese, copper, iodine, zinc, cobalt, fluoride, chromium, molybdenum, silicon, boron, and selenium.

Phytonutrients

Phytonutrients are substances found in plants that provide health benefits when included in a plant-based lifestyle. These powerful compounds may contain antioxidant, anti-carcinogen, and anti-inflammatory properties and can enhance immunity, repair DNA damage, and alter estrogen metabolism. Categories of phytonutrients include beta carotenes, lycopene, lutein, resveratrol, anthocyanins, and isoflavones and can be found in fruits and vegetables representing the colors of the rainbow.

AN APPLE A DAY...

Apples provide a rich source of phytochemicals which are linked to a reduction in heart disease, cancer, asthma, diabetes, and lowering cholesterol. They contain the 2nd highest level of antioxidants among common fruits

SCIENCE-BASED

TRUTH BEHIND VITAMIN D & CALCIUM

Plants Do a Body Good!

Vitamin D is very important for calcium absorption and bone growth. It also plays a role in immune function and serves as an anti-inflammatory. The media has pounded the importance of Vitamin D and calcium through the consumption of dairy products. This could not be further from the truth. Dairy products fortified with calcium and Vitamin D may actually decrease the calcium available for bone growth and maintenance. Why may this be so? Because dairy products are acidic to our bodies. As a response to their acidic nature, when our body detects changes in pH it releases neutralizing substances to bring it back to balance. One of these substances is suspected to be the calcium in our bones. So basically, dairy may not do a body good, it may actually do a body harm by depleting our calcium reserves and causing the exact opposite of what we erroneously believed it was doing - building up our bones.

What Is So Good About Antioxidants?

Antioxidants are substances that inhibit the oxidation of another molecule like oxygen. It is true that we need oxygen to live, but oxygen itself is a highly reactive compound that, if left to its own devices, inflicts havoc in our bodies. When a substance oxidizes, it produces free radicals which are the suspects in helping to cause diseases such as cancer, heart disease, Alzheimer's, arthritis, and a host of other ailments. It is a lot like having a bunch of tiny, rubber balls bouncing around in your vessels, hitting cells, organs, muscles, and tissues.

Antioxidants prevent this damage from occurring, but where do they come from? There are two sources of antioxidants, those naturally occurring in our bodies and in the foods we eat (for example, Vitamin A, C, E) and secondly, in industrially sourced antioxidants such as supplements, food additives, and preservatives.

Oxidative damage in DNA can cause cancer. Several antioxidant enzymes contained in whole, plant-based foods like berries, greens, peppers, carrots, and other brightly colored foods can protect DNA from oxidative stress. It is important to include a wide variety of these foods in your daily meals.

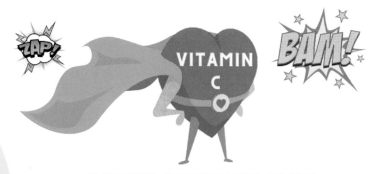

VITAMIN GUIDE

VITAMIN	VISION	SKIN	NERVES	CELLS	IMMUNE	ANTI-OXIDANT	BONE MUSCLE
Vitamin A	✓	✓			✓	✓	✓
Vitamin B2	✓	✓					
Vitamin B6				✓			
Vitamin B12			✓	✓			
Vitamin C					✓	✓	
Vitamin D							✓
Vitamin E				✓		✓	
Vitamin K				✓			
Folic Acid				✓			
Biotin				✓			

MINERAL GUIDE

FUNCTION

MINERAL	CLEANUP	NERVES	BLOOD CELLS	IMMUNE	DNA	HEART	MUSCLE BONE TEETH
Calcium		✓	✓			✓	✓
Chromium			✓				
Copper	✓	✓	✓				
Iron		✓	✓				
Magnesium		✓	✓			✓	✓
Manganese		✓	✓				✓
Molybdenum	✓			✓			✓
Potassium						✓	✓
Sodium		✓				✓	✓
Zinc			✓	✓	✓		

Whole Food Plant-Based 20

Chapter Eight

TIMING IS EVERYTHING

• •

Habits, Routines, Traditions, and Mindfulness

Habits, routines, and traditions—all things we are comfortable with, kind of like old comfy shoes. Sometimes, we hate to have to give them up and break in new ones. However, those same habits, routines, and traditions may not be what is best for us. They may not come from a good place or maybe we just have not given much thought to where they came from originally.

61

You may have gotten so used to them they have become second nature—no questioning involved. For many of us, habits and routines are part of our daily fabric. You wake up at a certain time each morning, you go to bed at a regular time, you eat specific foods for breakfast, lunch, and dinner. You may drive the same way to work each day. These are examples of regular routines.

Habits & Routines

In order to be successful in eating healthy, whole foods, you will begin to create new habits. What exactly is a habit? According to a 2012 study, "habits are actions that are triggered automatically in response to contextual cues that have been associated with their performance." [1] For example, putting your seatbelt on (action) whenever you get into a car (contextual cue) or washing your hands (action) whenever you use the restroom (contextual cue) are examples of habits. Your brain likes habits because they are predictable and efficient. Habits don't require much thought once they are ingrained and let the brain off the hook to focus on other things.

Establishing a new habit takes planning and attention. It is estimated that it takes anywhere from 20 days to three months to get into a new groove. [2] Certain habits take longer than others to change, especially if the said habit that you want to change brings pleasure, like eating. Awareness of your habits and

> In order to be successful in eating healthy, whole foods, you will begin to create new habits.

understanding them is a step in the right direction when you are trying to break or change a habit.

It is important to remember that each person is unique in their ability to adopt new habits or change old ones. There is no one size that fits all. Doing the same thing every day isn't for everyone. Even as you adopt a WFPB20 way of living, each one of you will start a little differently and continue in a slightly different way. That's all okay.

Whichever way you follow, remember the basis for WFPB20, a whole food plant-based diet is the healthiest lifestyle for your wellbeing, and keep this as your mantra. Adopting a new way, a healthier way, a whole-food, plant-based way, will lead you on the path to greater health and wellness. WFPB20 will get you jump-started in a new, healthy direction with guidance and resources for you to be successful.

Traditions

Traditions are frequently aligned with food. Memories of our childhood, holidays, special occasions, and celebrations—special foods are typically served during these gatherings. Our brains are wired to associate turkey with Thanksgiving, cake with birthdays, ice cream with summer outings, and hamburgers and hotdogs for baseball games or cookouts. WFPB20 will help you establish new, healthy ways of making celebratory foods, thus making new traditions. You don't forget the old traditions—keep those beautiful memories—but now you can make new ones to add to those past experiences. By being mindful of your actions and behaviors, you can move towards a healthier, more vibrant you.

Mindfulness

How do we become more mindful? Mindfulness is the state of being aware of your thoughts, emotions, feelings—both physically and mentally. In order to change your life patterns, you have to be mindful of what constitutes your habits, routines, and traditions. Where do they come from? Why do you have them? Do they bring you happiness, joy, stress, displeasure, indifference? Stop and pause for a moment and think about them. You will need brainpower to do this. You want to open up space in your mind and encourage freedom in that space to make a different decision. The power is in you, but you first have to allow it to happen. Look at these as objectively as you can. Take one at a time and give your attention to it.

Mindful Exercise

Is there one thing that you eat that you think may not be the healthiest for you? For example, do you put dairy-based cream in your coffee/tea because that is the way you have always had your coffee or tea? Can you think of another way to drink your coffee/tea that does not include a dairy-based product? Can you think about the effects of dairy on your health? Can you imagine if you eliminated that one thing and think about the health benefits you gain? Work your way through a series of exercises like this. Personalize them. Train your brain. It takes practice, but it works. You can use mindfulness to take you further down the road to better health and wellness.

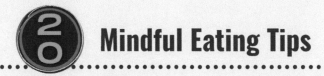 **Mindful Eating Tips**

1. Eat slowly with focus.

2. Eat only when you feel true hunger cues.

3. Eat until almost full—pay attention to your stomach cues.

4. Notice the colors of the food that you are eating.

5. Take in the smell of your food and connect it with happiness.

6. Sense the texture of the food you are eating.

7. Note triggers for eating like emotions or physical state.

8. Think about your health while eating.

9. Don't dwell on negativity if you eat something not healthy—let those feelings go.

10. Imagine disease retreating when eating healthy.

11. Serve your food on your favorite plate or bowl.

12. Eat with chopsticks to slow down the process.

13. Try eating with your opposite hand.

14. Eat while blindfolded and engage all of your senses.

15. Notice how your body feels after each meal—journal your feelings and track which foods bring you joy.

16. Be thankful for the food on your plate—say a mantra.

17. Take small bites of your food—savoring each one.

18. Chew each bite and notice the layers of tastes and textures.

19. Serve small portions of food and replenish until almost full.

20. Acknowledge your emotions before you begin to eat.

Chapter Nine

BECOME AN INGREDIENT DETECTIVE

· ·

Navigating the Product Label Jungle

It is a jungle out there when trying to discern what is actually in a product that you are buying or consuming. Nothing is worse than finding out the food that you have been eating under the guise of "healthy" contains the exact ingredients you have been trying to avoid.

For the most part, ingredients

are listed in the order of presence. For example, the first ingredient listed for any food typically is the main ingredient and makes up the greatest percentage of that particular food. The ingredients following are present in lesser and lesser amounts as the list progresses.

Many foods have unsuspecting ingredients, so you have to be extra vigilant and not take anything for granted. Who would have thought that spices have added oils or that non-dairy creamer has dairy in it? Or that orange juice can contain fish oils? When following a WFPB20 lifestyle, you will want to avoid animal products including dairy, oils, most sugars, possibly gluten, and other potentially harmful ingredients. This approach seems pretty straight forward, but it is actually very complex. The reason for this is that ingredients that you may not want are listed under a variety of names making this a more difficult task than imagined. In addition, sometimes, if ingredients make up a low percentage or are below a minimum value, they are not listed even if they are contained in the product.

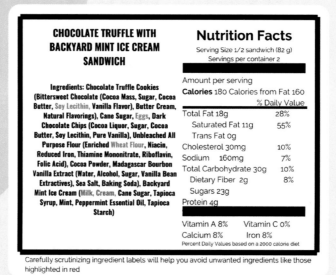

CHOCOLATE TRUFFLE WITH BACKYARD MINT ICE CREAM SANDWICH

Ingredients: Chocolate Truffle Cookies (Bittersweet Chocolate (Cocoa Mass, Sugar, Cocoa Butter, Soy Lecithin, Vanilla Flavor), Butter Cream, Natural Flavorings), Cane Sugar, Eggs, Dark Chocolate Chips (Cocoa Liquor, Sugar, Cocoa Butter, Soy Lecithin, Pure Vanilla), Unbleached All Purpose Flour (Enriched Wheat Flour, Niacin, Reduced Iron, Thiamine Mononitrate, Riboflavin, Folic Acid), Cocoa Powder, Madagascar Bourbon Vanilla Extract (Water, Alcohol, Sugar, Vanilla Bean Extractives), Sea Salt, Baking Soda), Backyard Mint Ice Cream (Milk, Cream, Cane Sugar, Tapioca Syrup, Mint, Peppermint Essential Oil, Tapioca Starch)

Nutrition Facts

Serving Size 1/2 sandwich (82 g)
Servings per container 2

Amount per serving

Calories 180 Calories from Fat 160

	% Daily Value
Total Fat 18g	28%
Saturated Fat 11g	55%
Trans Fat 0g	
Cholesterol 30mg	10%
Sodium 160mg	7%
Total Carbohydrate 30g	10%
Dietary Fiber 2g	8%
Sugars 23g	
Protein 4g	

Vitamin A 8%	Vitamin C 0%
Calcium 8%	Iron 8%

Percent Daily Values based on a 2000 calorie diet

Carefully scrutinizing ingredient labels will help you avoid unwanted ingredients like those highlighted in red

Claims made on packaging can be misleading. For example, non-dairy does not mean that the product is milk-free. Under the FDA guidelines, it can still contain casein, which is the component of milk that is linked to cancer. Here are a few culprits to look out for:

- **Bagels/Bread:** Many bread products contain an amino acid known as L-cysteine, which is used as a softening agent. L-cysteine is derived naturally from either human hair or poultry feathers or can be synthetically prepared.
- **Non-dairy creamer:** Although it has non-dairy in its name, many such creamers contain casein, a protein derived from milk.
- **Omega-3 products:** There are some products with labels that boast their heart-healthy ingredients that contain omega-3 fatty acids derived from fish. For example, a popular heart healthy orange juice label lists tilapia, sardines, and anchovy as ingredients.
- **Peanuts:** Some brands of peanuts, especially dry roasted, also contain gelatin because the substance helps salt and other spices adhere to the nuts.
- **Sugar:** There are over 56 names for sugar! Sugar isn't naturally white, so manufacturers process it using bone char, which is made from the bones of cattle. To avoid sugar filtered with bone char, purchase unrefined sugar, or buy from brands that don't use bone-char filters.
- **Refried beans:** Many canned refried beans are made with hydrogenated lard, so check labels to ensure you're buying vegetarian beans.
- **Tortillas:** You would think that something as basic as a tortilla would be safe territory but think again. Many brands contain lard and/or oil along with other additives. Flour tortillas are the main culprits, but

corn tortillas can also contain unhealthy ingredients.

- **Vanilla-flavored foods:** Beware of "natural flavorings." Although not common, some foods are flavored with castoreum, a beaver anal secretion. The FDA classifies it as "generally recognized as safe," and it is most often used in baked goods as a vanilla substitute, but it's also been used in alcoholic beverages, puddings, ice cream, candy, and chewing gum.

- **Worcestershire sauce**: This popular sauce is made with anchovies, but vegetarian-friendly brands are available.

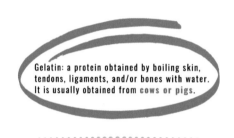

Gelatin: a protein obtained by boiling skin, tendons, ligaments, and/or bones with water. It is usually obtained from cows or pigs.

Fish in OJ?

Ingredients: 100% Pure pasteurized orange juice, fish oil (anchovy and sardine oils)*, fish gelatin (tilapia)*, sodium ascorbate* and citric acid*.

*Ingredient not found in regular orange juice.

Contains tilapia, sardine and anchovy.

Contains orange juice from U.S. and Brazil.

›◉MEG-3®
trust the source ®

MEG-3® and trust the source® are trademarks of Ocean Nutrition Canada Ltd., Dartmouth, Nova Scotia, Canada B2Y 4T6

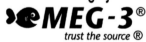

Different Names Used For Sugar

1. Agave Nectar
2. Molasses
3. Cane Sugar
4. Date Sugar
5. Lactose
6. Carob Syrup
7. Brown Sugar
8. Corn Syrup
9. Caramel
10. Glucose
11. Fructose
12. Maltose
13. Rice Syrup
14. Sucrose
15. Dextrose
16. Evaporated Cane Juice
17. Maltodextrin
18. Honey
19. High Fructose Corn Syrup
20. Fruit Juice Concentrate

Chapter Ten

WE BEGIN

Getting Your House in Order—Pantry, Stock & Kitchen Tools

Timing

Sometimes timing is everything. Catching a bus or a train, baking a cake, or even crossing the street. When it comes to making changes to your lifestyle, especially when it comes to the food you eat, you must allow sufficient time to adjust. Reset your expectations that this is all not going to happen instantaneously. It will take work on your part. But like any good plan, the time and consideration you put into it in the beginning, will pay big dividends in the end. Keep in mind that you will need to adjust your menu planning, your grocery shopping, your food supplies, your habits, your taste buds, and your mindset in order to be successful. For most people, this does not happen overnight. WFPB20 is set on a 20-day cycle. You can cycle through this once or 100 times. However many times you personally need to get moving in the right direction is the perfect number of times. Remember this is all about YOUR journey.

Pantry Raid

No matter where you store all of your food supplies, in order to be successful in making changes to your daily foods you must be vigilant in removing all of the bad players from your living space. In order to do this, you have to identify the bad players. In Chapter Nine, we learned how to read ingredient labels and what to look out for. We will now put that to the test in your kitchen. Reading the label on every package, bottle, can, bag, and box you have that contains food is the surest way to identify the bad players right off of the bat.

Your first step will be to remove everything from your storage areas and place it nearby. This will look really messy at first, but there is a method to this madness. Next, go through each item to check the labels for animal products, oils, sugars, additives, and other harmful ingredients. Remove any products that contain these items by either tossing them in the trash or donating them. They cannot go back into your storage area because they will derail your efforts if you keep them within reach. You will want to repeat this process for your refrigerator and freezer. Clean it all out.

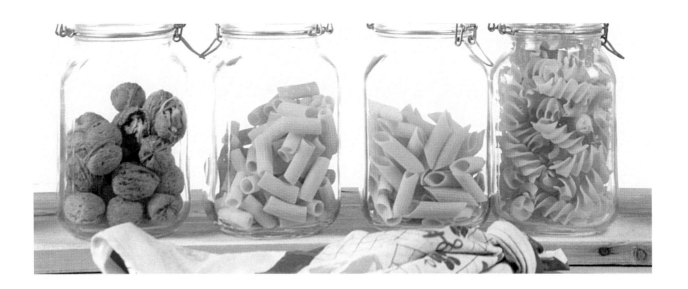

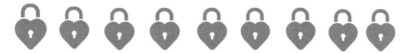

CREATE A SAFE SPACE

Whether you live in an apartment, garage, basement, condo, or mansion - the first step to success is ensuring you have a safe environment free of foods that will trip you up. If you share this space with others, then setting up a specific location where you store your stuff will go a long way to help to keep you on track. A handy tip to help secure your space is to use blue painter's tape. You can use it to mark off a section in your refrigerator or simply mark your food with a piece of it.

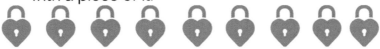

Take Stock of Your Stock

Now that you have gotten rid of the products with the less than desirable ingredients, you are safely left with compliant foods. You will want to return these to your storage area in an organized fashion. Grouping them according to their classification (e.g. pasta, beans, canned goods, seasonings, flavorings) will help to quickly assess what you have on hand, figure out what is running low, and find items when you are cooking.

This will help you in your meal planning and preparation as well as in making your grocery shopping list.

You can keep either an electronic or written record of what you have so that you can access it any time while you are away from home. This makes planning meals on the run a cinch. No guessing at the grocery store and it can save you money in the long run by not buying duplicate products.

Getting Down to the Basics

Eating a plant-based diet does not have to be complicated. The simpler the better. At first, your shopping list will be crowded with items that you either do not have on hand or are unfamiliar with. That is okay. It will get easier as time goes on and you continue on this path of healthy living. By following the list of 20 of the right stuff, you will make your initial foray a little bit easier. You don't need to invest your dollars in a ton of fresh fruits and veggies at first. Frozen varieties do just fine when you are starting out. You can throw in some bananas, grapes, and apples on your first grocery trip if you enjoy eating these fresh.

The ingredients listed here are versatile enough that you can prepare a bunch of meals with just these combinations. You can compile your shopping list once you have selected what you are going to make for the first week. Cross-reference what you have and what you will need for your grocery list.

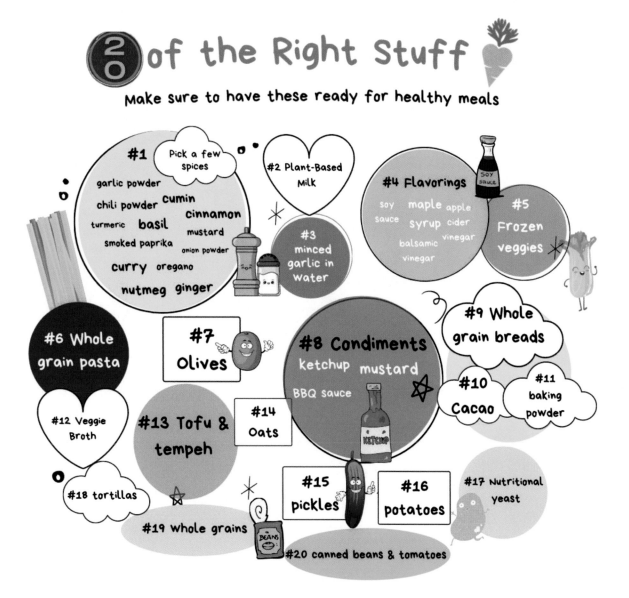

20 of the Right Stuff

Make sure to have these ready for healthy meals

#1 Pick a few spices
garlic powder
chili powder cumin
turmeric basil cinnamon
smoked paprika mustard
onion powder
curry oregano
nutmeg ginger

#2 Plant-Based Milk

#3 minced garlic in water

#4 Flavorings
soy sauce maple apple
syrup cider
balsamic vinegar
vinegar

#5 Frozen veggies

#6 Whole grain pasta

#7 Olives

#8 Condiments
ketchup mustard
BBQ sauce

#9 Whole grain breads

#10 Cacao

#11 baking powder

#12 Veggie Broth

#13 Tofu & tempeh

#14 Oats

#15 pickles

#16 potatoes

#17 Nutritional yeast

#18 tortillas

#19 whole grains

#20 canned beans & tomatoes

The Right Tools for the Job

For kitchen utensils and equipment, you don't have to go out and buy anything right away. You can make do with a sharp knife and a can opener if you want to really keep it simple. However, here is a list for your reference that you can review and determine what items will fit your cooking style and needs.

 TOP Kitchen & Cooking Favs

1. **High-speed blender**—when you are making smoothies or nut butters, a high-speed blender does the trick. Vitamix is the king, but there are others like the Ninja blender line, that will also do the job and not cost a small fortune.

2. **Food processor**—mixing fillings, prepping, and chopping up ingredients into smaller pieces is conveniently done with a food processor. These come in all shapes and sizes. It is recommended that you read the reviews online before you purchase one.

3. **Electric pressure cooker and/or slow cooker**—a real time-saver in the kitchen for soups, chilis, stews, pasta, beans, and grains. Modern-day pressure cookers are outfitted with many safety features so there is no need to worry about exploding pots on your stove.

4. **Paring knife and chef's knife**—sharp knives are the way to go when you spend time preparing fresh foods. Try the Westhof for your Chef's prep knife or ceramic knives from Cuisinart. Buy, and regularly use, a honing steel rod to keep your knives sharp.

5. **Hand-held can opener**— For back to basics you can try the Kuhn Rikon Safety hand-operated can opener. It removes the lid with no sharp edges. Very old school but it works.

6. **Vegetable peeler**—any peeler will do although there are multi-purpose peelers, spiralizers, and shredders out there.

7. **Colander**— not just for draining pasta but also great for rinsing and draining veggies, beans, and fruits. Get several in different sizes depending on your need.

8. **Cookware**—you will need a couple of different size pots, flat pans for grilling, and a soup pot. Check out the high-grade stainless-steel versions. For health reasons, avoid the nonstick surface cookware.

9. **Measuring cups**—for liquids and solids try glass Pyrex measuring cups and stainless-steel cups.

10. **Measuring spoons**—pick your favorite and you can never have too many sets.

11. **Cutting boards**—try a variety of sizes and materials and see what you like the best.

12. **Baking pans**—flat baking pans, and cake and loaf pans are great for roasting veggies, baking cornbread, muffins, and cakes.

13. **Parchment paper**—a wonderful tool for nonstick baking and cooking plus no oil needed.

14. **Glass storage containers**—avoid chemicals leaching into your foods by using glass storage containers.

15. **Mixing bowls**—a set of different size bowls can aid when prepping multiple dishes.

16. **Zester/Grater**—when you want to add a little citrus zest to your dishes or need to grate chocolate or nutmeg this tool comes in handy.

17. **Cake tester**—a great tool to test baked goods for doneness or toothpicks work just as well.

18. **Mason jars**—perfect for storing dressings, sauces, overnight oats, grains, legumes, nuts, seeds, fruits, veggies, and more.

19. **Oven mitts**—nothing like a good quality oven mitt to protect your hands

20. **Citrus juicer**—handy for squeezing lemons, oranges, limes, and other citrus fruits.

••

Chapter Eleven

BATCH COOKING & PREP

Planning ahead is really the key to success in most things in life, especially when it comes to adopting WFPB20. With a little effort and prep work you can make eating healthy, quick and easy, which ensures your success. Preparing meals ahead of time and not waiting until you are desperately hungry goes a long way too.

What is Batch Cooking?

Batch cooking is the planning and preparation of a variety of multi-serving meals all at once, and then either refrigerating or freezing labeled portions for future meals.

The first steps in batch cooking include the planning of your meals, gathering the recipes, and shopping for the ingredients. You can decide how many meals you will want to prep for your days or the week ahead. You get to tailor your batch cooking sessions according to your needs and wants. Choosing a day and time that works for your schedule can keep you on track. However, if your schedule is fluid and ever-changing then your batch cooking session can be flexible from week to week.

If you have never batch cooked before, then take it slow. Choose one or two meals at first to see how it goes. For example, you could decide just to prep your breakfasts and two different recipes for dinner. You choose Overnight Oats for your breakfast all week, and a soup and chili for your two dinner recipes. Both of the dinner recipes can be eaten two or three nights each. You could also include them as your lunch choice for the week. You change up how you serve them as well. For instance, if you make chili, you can serve it traditionally in a bowl with some cornbread on the side. The next time, you serve it over a baked potato. Or you can wrap it in a tortilla for a quick lunch. For the soup you chose, you can serve it for dinner with bread and a side veggie, and you could serve it for lunch along with a side salad. In this scenario, your batch cooking session could take anywhere from an hour to a couple of hours depending on how complex or simple your recipes are. At the end of the session, you have your breakfasts, dinners and lunches prepped for the week ahead. With simple reheating and assembly, you have a week of successes all ready for you.

Tips and Ideas for Batch Cooking

1. Bake a bunch of potatoes: sweet, red and/or Russet potatoes—they can be used for meals and snacks during the week.

2. Cut up veggies like carrots, celery, peppers, and cukes and store for snacking or salads.

3. Prepare one of your favorite dips like hummus or black bean dip. They make great snacks, dressings, or toppings on tortillas and potatoes.

4. Prep a dressing for your weekly salad.

5. Fill 5 mason jars with overnight oat mix for breakfast.

6. Bake up a batch of vegan muffins for on-the-go breakfast or snacks.

7. Cook up a batch of whole grains like rice or quinoa.

8. Cook up a batch of dried beans and freeze in 1 ½ cup portions (equals one can).

9. Wash a mixture of greens and store in an airtight container with a paper towel in the refrigerator.

10. Make a double serving of a soup, stew, chili, or casserole and freeze half in labeled glass containers.

11. Fix a batch of veggie burgers and freeze for later.

12. To save time in chopping, buy frozen chopped veggies.

13. Mix smoothie ingredients together ahead of time and store in the freezer.

14. Buy frozen fruit to ensure you always have fruit available for breakfast, smoothies, and salads.

15. Save time and tears and buy frozen chopped onions.

16. Wash fresh cilantro and parsley and keep in a jar with water in the refrigerator. Just snip off what you need without having to stop and wash.

17. Fill pint mason jars with chopped fresh veggies, cooked legumes and grains, and diced raw sweet potatoes; cover tightly and store in the refrigerator. Quickly add to dishes throughout the week.

18. Freeze ripe bananas by removing skins, slicing them into chunks, and laying them on a flat plate without touching and sticking them in the freezer for an hour or so. Then place frozen chunks into a freezer bag or container. Use in smoothies and desserts.

19. Prep a fresh pitcher of tea or flavored water (cucumber, orange slices) and store in the refrigerator for a refreshing after-noon drink.

20. Prepare a batch of "nice cream" and freeze it for future desserts.

PRESSURE COOKER CHEATS
Pressure cookers are a safe, fast,
and healthy way to make WFPB meals
(INGREDIENTS ARE UNCOOKED)

INGREDIENT	AMT	H2O	Time (min)
black beans	1 cup	3 cups	45
white rice	1 cup	1 cup	7
quinoa	1 cup	1.5 cups	1+10NPR*
steel-cut oats	3/4 cup	1 3/4 cups	4
sweet potatoes	4-5	1 cup	22
spaghetti squash	1/2	1 cup	7

*NPR - natural pressure release

Embrace Your Hunger. We have been ingrained to think that hunger pains are a bad thing. They are the signal to the brain that all of the food you have eaten has been digested and used and now it is time to provide more nourishment. If you can wait it out just a bit you will train your body to utilize its stored reserves. Observe how you can actually get past those hunger pangs and spread a little more time out in between meals. It is the fast track to losing weight faster if that is your thing.

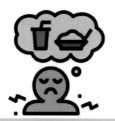

Chapter Twelve

HEALTHY SUBSTITUTIONS

• •

 ## Substitutes for NO OIL Cooking

1. Use water and/or veggie broth for stove-top sauté.
2. Replace oil with parchment paper when baking foods in the oven.
3. Season vegetables first when roasting and spray lightly with water while cooking.
4. Before cooking, flavor your veggies and other foods with oil-free marinades.
5. Caramelize onions and shallots using water to deglaze the pan.
6. Substitute applesauce for oil in recipes.
7. Sub out oil with flaxseed.
8. Use prune or date puree for oil in baking recipes.
9. Use silicone baking mats and bakeware for your baked goods.
10. Blend in white beans into sauces and dressings to replace the oil.

11. Tofu is another good substitute for oil in dressings and sauces.
12. Balsamic vinegar in a variety of flavors can be used for dressings, sauces, and marinades.
13. Mustards add depth and spice to dishes in lieu of oils.
14. A variety of fruits like berries, apples, and bananas can be substitutes.
15. Tamari is flavorful and gives a nutty and umami edge to a dish.
16. Date syrup is a great enhancer to marinades, dressings, and sauces.
17. Pureed pumpkin adds wonderful moistness and creaminess to dishes.
18. Cooked cauliflower is another alternative and does not add any flavor, just texture.
19. Mashed avocado adds fat and creaminess.
20. Nuts, including cashews and peanuts, enhance sauces and texture.

· ·

Chapter Thirteen

EATING OUT & AWAY

• •

Whether you are new to a whole food plant-based way of eating or experienced, venturing outside of your home to have a meal can be intimidating. Even if you aren't new to this way of eating, eating out can still be fraught with stress. It really does not need to be. While you may not have as much control as you do when eating at home, with proper planning and flexibility, you can enjoy eating out with friends and family just like you did before you changed your diet. There may be times that you have to be flexible in the food options in that some foods may contain oil. For those more infrequent instances when you are eating out, give yourself permission to try your best, even if it is not perfect. Online resources like HappyCow.net and Vegman.org can help you navigate healthy eateries while out and about.

Tips for Eating Out the WFPB20 Way

1. Provide some input to the restaurant selection by using convenient online apps for finding vegan-friendly eateries.

2. Choose ethnic-based restaurants that have a wider appeal and offer something for everyone.

3. Call ahead to the restaurant and inquire about a vegan menu or options.

4. Eat something beforehand if the restaurant or event that you are attending has no vegan options.

5. Bring a small snack with you that you can indiscreetly eat at the restaurant if there are no options.

6. When you arrive, ask to speak to the waitstaff or chef before everyone orders to discuss your preferences.

7. When ordering, sometimes it is better to suggest to the waitstaff that you have an allergy to animal products and/or oil than to explain what veganism is all about.

8. Be polite and smile when discussing the menu and be as flexible as you can.

9. Ensure that you can make substitutions like avocado instead of cheese, or corn tortillas in place of flour tortillas.

10. Observe icons on the menu designating vegan, gluten-free, or vegetarian options.

11. Scan menu for sides, salads, and main course selections that can be modified in how they are cooked or served.

12. Japanese cuisine offerings include edamame, vegan sushi rolls, miso soups, rice, and veggie options—make sure you specify no fish sauce or egg.

13. Chinese cuisine may include spring rolls, noodle and rice dishes, steamed veggies without fish or oyster sauces.

14. For Thai food, there are a variety of curries, spring rolls, green mango salads, noodles, and rice dishes. Ensure the curry sauces are vegan and contain no fish.

15. Greek food has a lot to offer in terms of vegan options. These include hummus, falafel, salads, pita, eggplant, and grilled veggie wraps along with rice and veggies.

16. Classic steakhouse restaurants often have some of the best side options. For example: baked potatoes, steamed vegetables, fries (you may have to be flexible here), vegetarian chilis, BBQ tofu, and salads.

17. Indian restaurants have many options that include rice and vegetables, samosas, dal, chana masalas, and bread. Make sure that those dishes do not contain ghee or yogurt.

18. Italian dishes of pasta, marinara sauces, soups, pizzas, and salads can all be offered without meat and dairy.

19. Burger joints frequently offer vegetarian or vegan options featuring veggie or Beyond Meat or Impossible Burgers. You can also order all of the fixings without the meat and cheese.

20. If you are attending a private party, contact the host ahead of time and discuss food options for you. If there are none, then offer to bring something that meets your preferences and that can be shared.

WFBP20 on the Road

Whether you are traveling by plane, train or automobile, there are lots of ways to adequately prepare for the unexpected when it comes to eating WFPB. Here are a few tips:

- Pack fruit and cut up veggies along with hummus or other dips
- Carry overnight or instant oats and add water or milk
- Pack steamed potatoes along with mustard, ketchup, or salsa
- Popcorn, rice cakes with peanut butter, pretzels
- Prep sandwiches, wraps, or salads
- A thermos filled with soup, chili, or smoothies
- Nuts, raisins, almonds, whole sunflower seeds, or pistachio nuts
- Frozen water bottles to keep food cold and drink when thawed

Chapter Fourteen

LET'S EAT

• •

It's time to put what you learned to the test. WFPB20 is set up to provide you with a menu template that you can adapt and make your own. It provides breakfast ideas and recipes, interchangeable lunch and dinner recipes along with additional sauces, salads, snack, and dessert ideas. These recipes are very flexible for a reason. There is no one menu that fits everyone's time constraints, abilities, tastes, and preferences. The meals outlined here are intended to be repeated and eventually modified to suit your needs. This is a starting place for your WFPB20 journey.

Map out what appeals to you and what fits into your schedule when you begin the 20 days. The meals included have uncomplicated ingredients and instructions. Plus, ingredients are duplicated throughout so you can be the most efficient in your prep work. Wishing you a delicious 20 days and beyond!

KISS
Keep it simple silly!

Pick recipes you look forward to eating and that sound appealing.

2-3 prepared dishes can be recycled throughout your week keeping you out of the kitchen most nights.

Don't focus on what you cannot have but rather focus on what you CAN eat.

Prepare healthy snacks.

If you plan to be away from home for most of the day either at work or somewhere else pack more food than you can possibly eat in a day.

Desserts are a Good Thing. Plan to make some sweet rewards that are also healthy.

Set a time at night where the kitchen is closed. Drink tea, brush your teeth – have a mental close to your day.

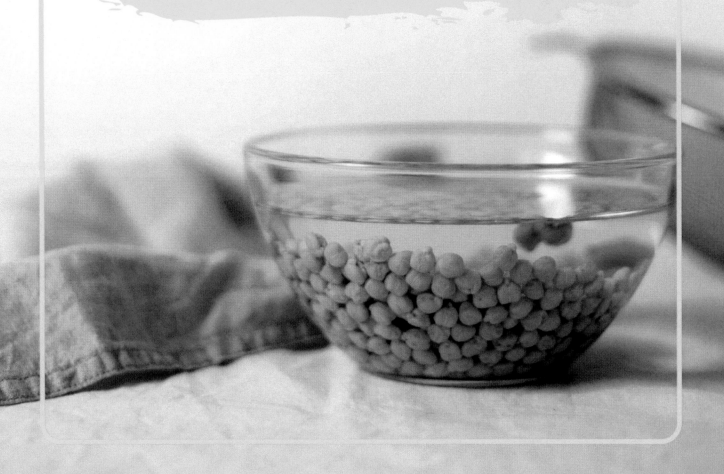

RECIPES

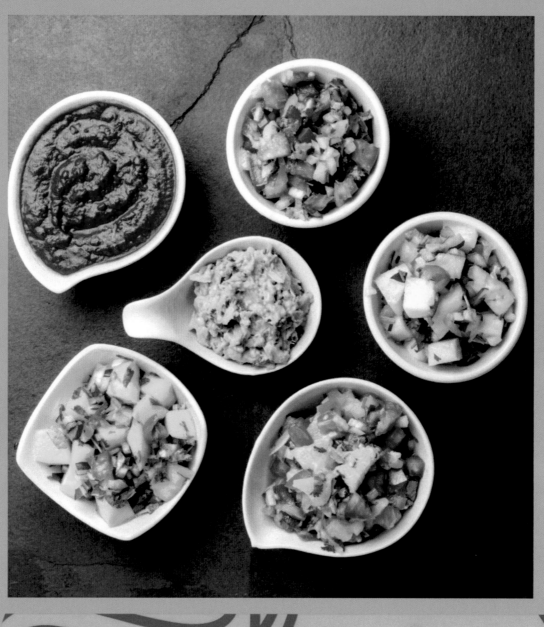

MAYONNAISE

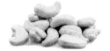

1 1/2 cups raw cashews, soaked in boiling water 1 hour+

2 tsp lemon juice

2 Tbs distilled white vinegar

1/8 tsp ground mustard seed

1/8 tsp fresh minced garlic

3/4 cup plus 1 Tbs water

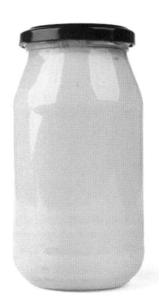

Place all ingredients into high-speed blender and blend until smooth. Place in glass jar with lid and put in refrigerator to thicken.

SOUR CREAM

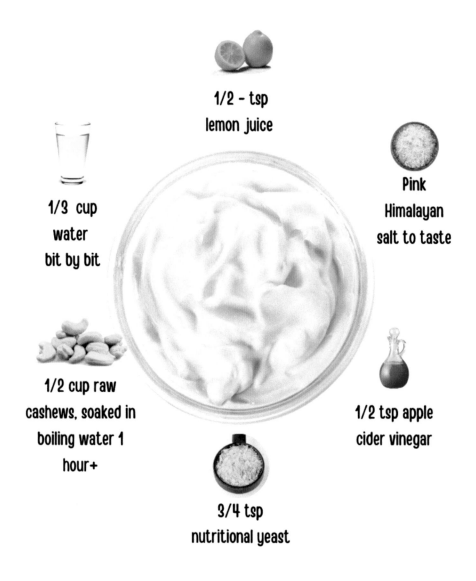

1/2 - tsp
lemon juice

1/3 cup
water
bit by bit

Pink
Himalayan
salt to taste

1/2 cup raw
cashews, soaked in
boiling water 1
hour+

1/2 tsp apple
cider vinegar

3/4 tsp
nutritional yeast

Combine all ingredients in Vitamix or high-speed blender, adding water bit by bit until completely smooth and at the desired consistency. Refrigerate to thicken.

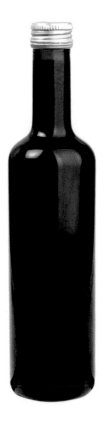

BALSAMIC GLAZE

Bring 2 cups of quality balsamic vinegar to boil over medium heat. Turn to simmer and cook until 1/2 cup remains and it is noticeably thicker (~20 minutes). Remove from heat, allow to cool and increase in thickness. Place in a covered glass container and store in refrigerator.

CREAMY ALFREDO SAUCE

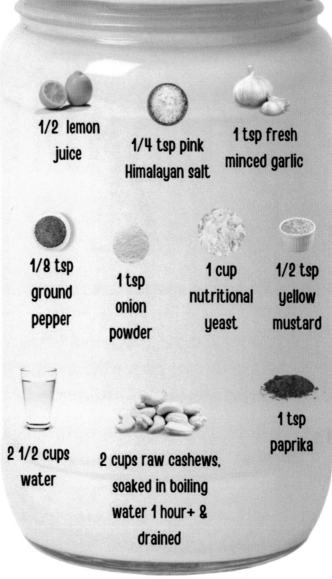

1/2 lemon juice

1/4 tsp pink Himalayan salt

1 tsp fresh minced garlic

1/8 tsp ground pepper

1 tsp onion powder

1 cup nutritional yeast

1/2 tsp yellow mustard

2 1/2 cups water

2 cups raw cashews, soaked in boiling water 1 hour+ & drained

1 tsp paprika

Mix drained cashews and water in a high-speed blender and blend until smooth. Add all remaining ingredients and blend until incorporated. Add water as needed for a creamy consistency. Place in glass jar with lid and refrigerate to thicken.

GUACAMOLE

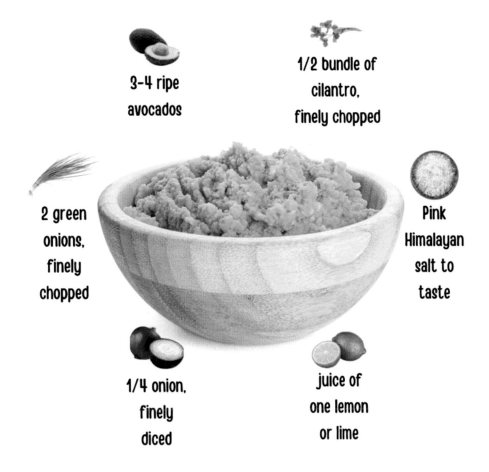

3-4 ripe
avocados

1/2 bundle of
cilantro,
finely chopped

2 green
onions,
finely
chopped

Pink
Himalayan
salt to
taste

1/4 onion,
finely
diced

juice of
one lemon
or lime

Finely chop or dice all ingredients and mix them in a bowl. Cut and add the avocados first mashing them with a fork. Add the juice of lemon or lime once mixed. Sprinkle with Himalayan salt.

1 cup
tomatoes

 1/2 red
onion,
diced

 1/2
bundle
of
cilantro,
finely
chopped

 Pink
Himalayan
salt to taste

 juice of
one
lemon
or lime

PICO DE GALLO

Finely chop or dice all ingredients and mix them in a bowl. Add the juice of lemon or lime once mixed. Sprinkle with Himalayan salt.

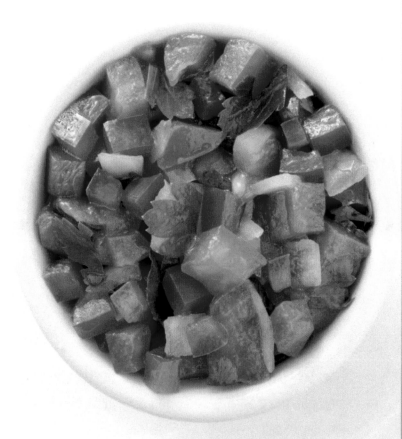

optional: green onions chopped and finely diced jalapeño pepper (flesh removed to make it less spicy)

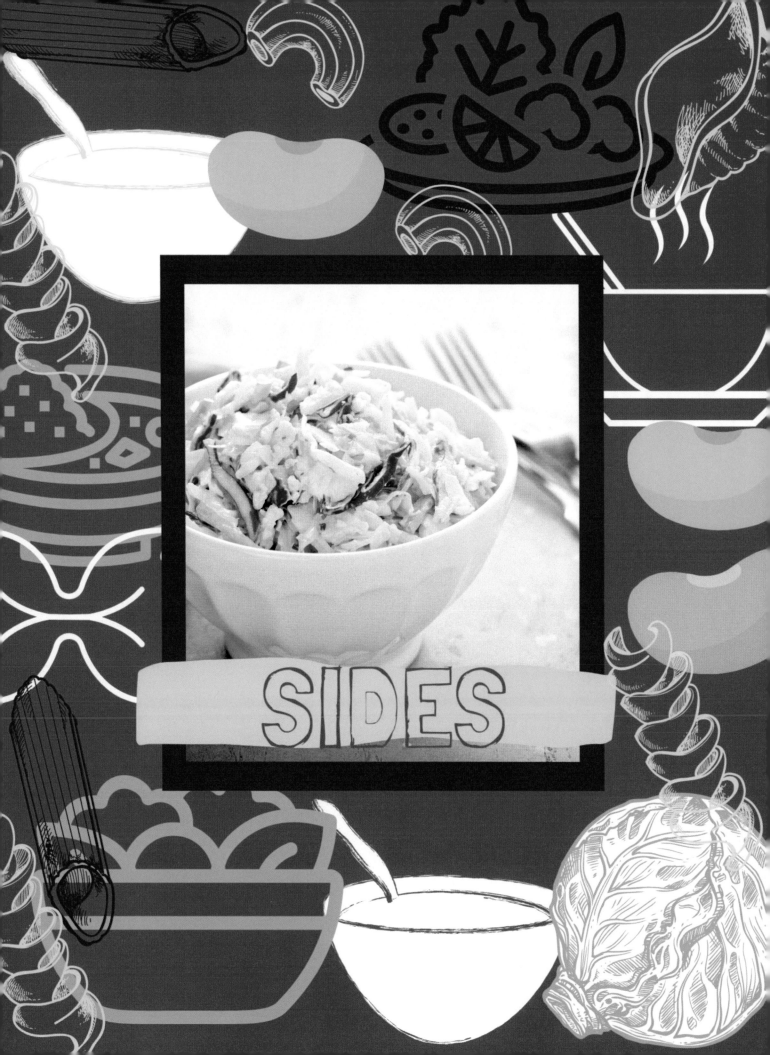

SIDES

1/2 small head cabbage, shredded

2 large carrots, shredded

1 medium jicama, shredded

juice of 2 limes

5-8 dashes ume plum vinegar

1/4 small head purple cabbage, shredded

1 large green apple, shredded

1 handful cilantro, chopped

Cashew Mayo (see recipe)

COLESLAW

In a large bowl combine all ingredients until well mixed. Garnish with toasted seeds (pumpkin, walnut, or sunflower). Serve immediately or store in an airtight container in the fridge for approximately 5-7 days. Enjoy!

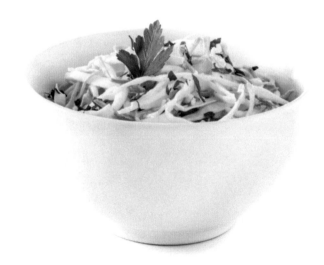

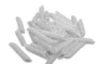

rice or
wheat
pasta

avocado

fresh basil or
parsley chopped

orange bell
pepper
chopped

olives

salt/pepper

PASTA SALAD

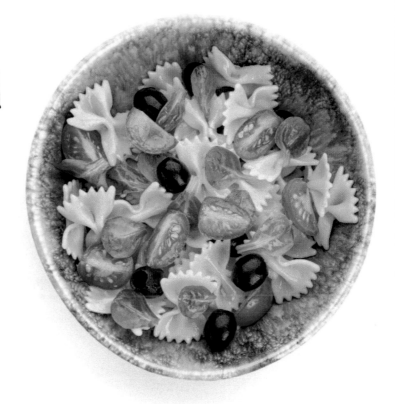

While boiling the pasta, chop all
vegetables. Mix in large bowl and
garnish with extra basil on top.

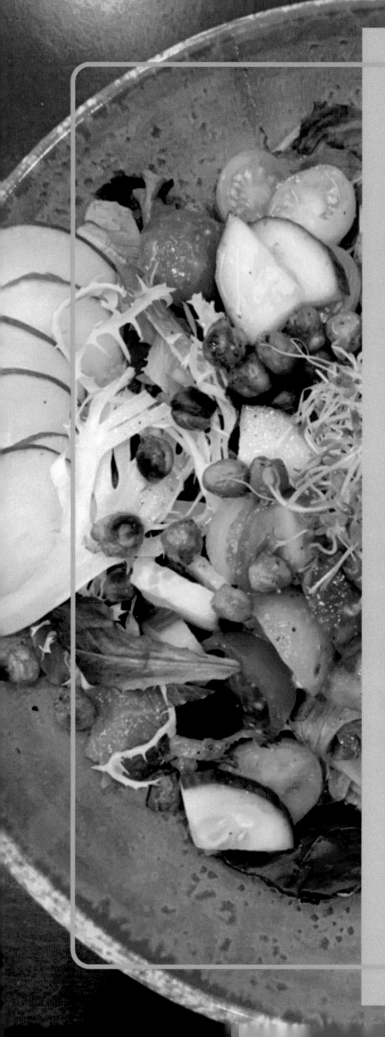

HIGH PROTEIN CROUTONS

1/2 tsp cinnamon

1/4 tsp cloves

1 tsp coriander

1 1/2 tsp turmeric

1/2 tsp ginger

2 tsp smoked paprika

1 Tbs cumin

1/8 tsp cayenne

1 tsp salt

4 Tbs maple syrup

1 tsp coconut aminos

2 cans chickpeas, drained

Preheat oven to 375°F. Line baking sheet with parchment paper. Drain and rinse chickpeas, pour into large bowl and stir in coconut aminos to coat. Make spice blend and stir into the chickpeas. Pour into single layer on the baking sheet and bake for 30 minutes, stirring half way through. Turn off oven and let sit for 1 hour until crispy. Place in glass jar with lid. Top on salads or enjoy as a snack.

EDAMAME & SWEET POTATO SALAD

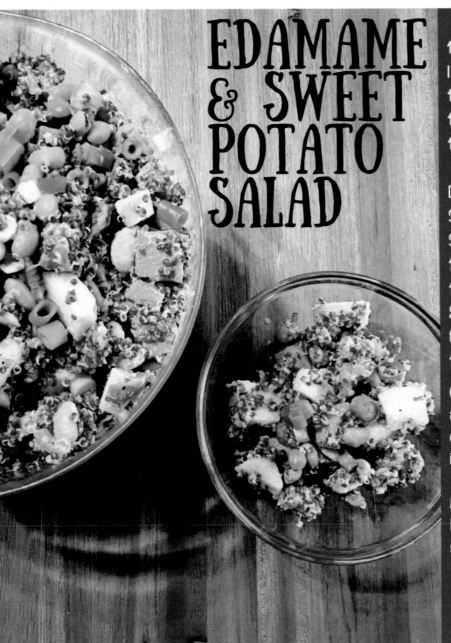

1 cup quinoa

1 cup jicama, chopped small

1 cup diced sweet potato (baked)

1 cup edamame, steamed

1/2 cup green onions, chopped

Dressing:

3 garlic cloves

3 Tbs maple syrup

1/4 cup white miso paste

1 cup tahini

2 Tbs tamari

fresh grated ginger

1/2 cup water

Chop sweet potato, season with salt and pepper, bake at 400°F for 20 min or until crisp. Set aside. Rinse quinoa & cook according to directions. Chop other ingredients while food is cooking.

Mix dressing in food processor. Combine all ingredients in a bowl, add dressing. Chill in fridge until ready to serve.

Oatmeal w/ Berries, Nuts, Cinnamon & Dates

Avocado Toast

Tofu Scramble

Smoothie

Overnight Oats with Fruit

Nut Butter and Banana

Tofu Scramble Taco's

Smoothie Bowl

Chia Seed Parfait with Fruit

Cubed Potatoes with Sautéed Mushrooms and Onions

Tofu Scramble Wrap with Spinach

Fruit and Vegan Yogurt

Sweet Potato with Hummus

Granola and Fruit

Cliff Bar

Banana and Peanut Butter

Garbanzo Bean Crepe

Sautéed Veggies with Tofu Cubes

Pancakes

Waffles

AVOCADO TOAST

whole grain toast

ripe mashed avocado

sprouts, seeds

sliced tomato, jalapenos

smoked paprika, salt & pepper, garlic granules, balsamic glaze, salsa

Build your own. You can substitute hummus for the avocado

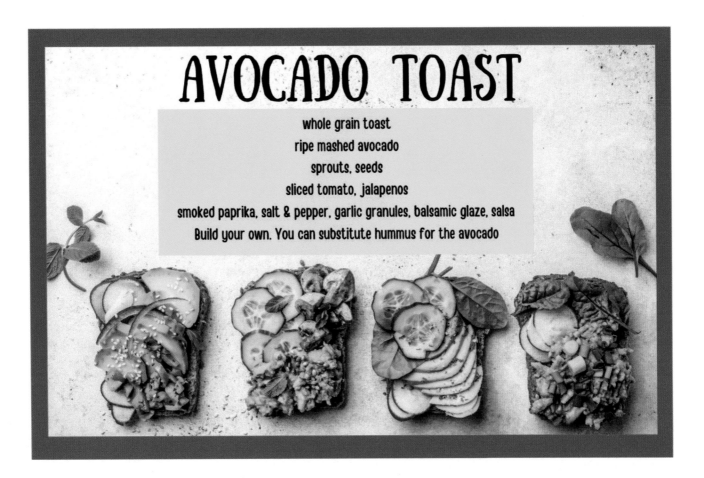

OVERNIGHT PARFAITS

- use a glass jar with an airtight lid
- add 1/3 cup organic rolled oats
- add ~1 cup plant-based milk
- add seeds: flax, chia, hemp, sesame
- add crushed nuts: walnuts, almonds, pecans, pistachios, coconut

NOTE: add all toppings as preferred and to taste

- add dried fruit: raisins, dates, cranberries, gogi
- add spices: cinnamon, cardamom, nutmeg
- add flavorings: date or maple syrup, cacao, vanilla, nut butters
- shake and leave in the refrigerator overnight
- top with fresh fruit in morning

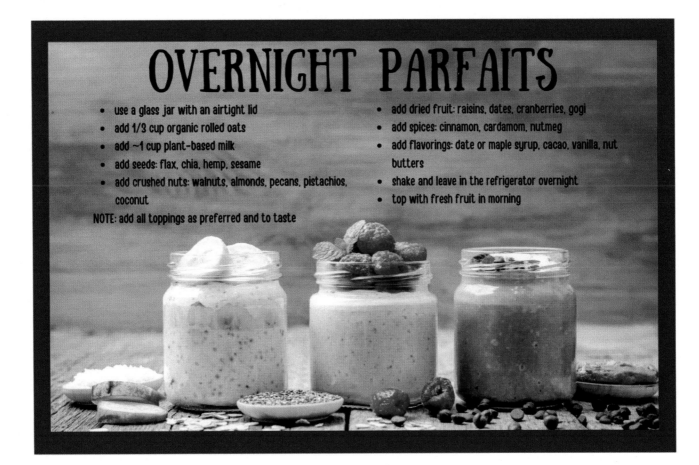

SMOOTHIE BOWLS

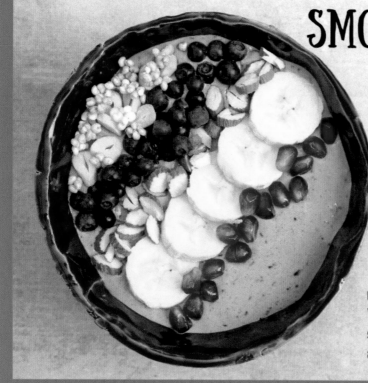

- Start with your favorite smoothie mixture of fruits and veggies (e.g. bananas, blueberries, mango, pineapple, spinach, kale) prepared in a blender, but add less milk to make it thicker.
- Pour mixture into a wide bowl.
- Top with whole fresh berries (blueberries, raspberries, blackberries, or strawberries),
- Sprinkle with walnuts, almonds, or pistachios.
- Add chia, pumpkin, or sesame seeds.
- Add some slices of fruit like banana, peaches, or apples.
- Add some toasted oats or coconut.

NOTES:

You can use frozen fruit and veggies for the smoothie and fresh fruit for the bowl. Mix it up and add your favorites to make it your own.

BREKKIE TACOS

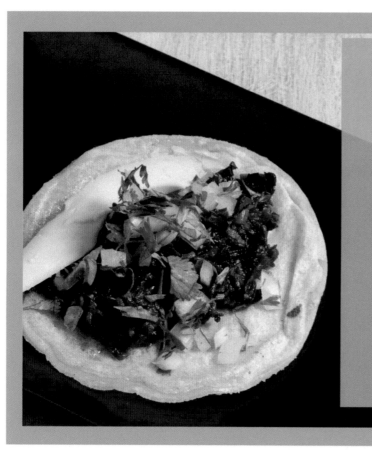

Load up tortillas, (corn or flour, soft or hard) with refried or seasoned beans or scrambled tofu, tomatoes, avocado, greens, and top it all off with sour cream and salsa.

Variations: cubed roasted russet or sweet potatoes, tempeh bacon, hummus, olives, red onions, pickled radishes or jalapeños, shredded cabbage, sauted mushroom & peppers.

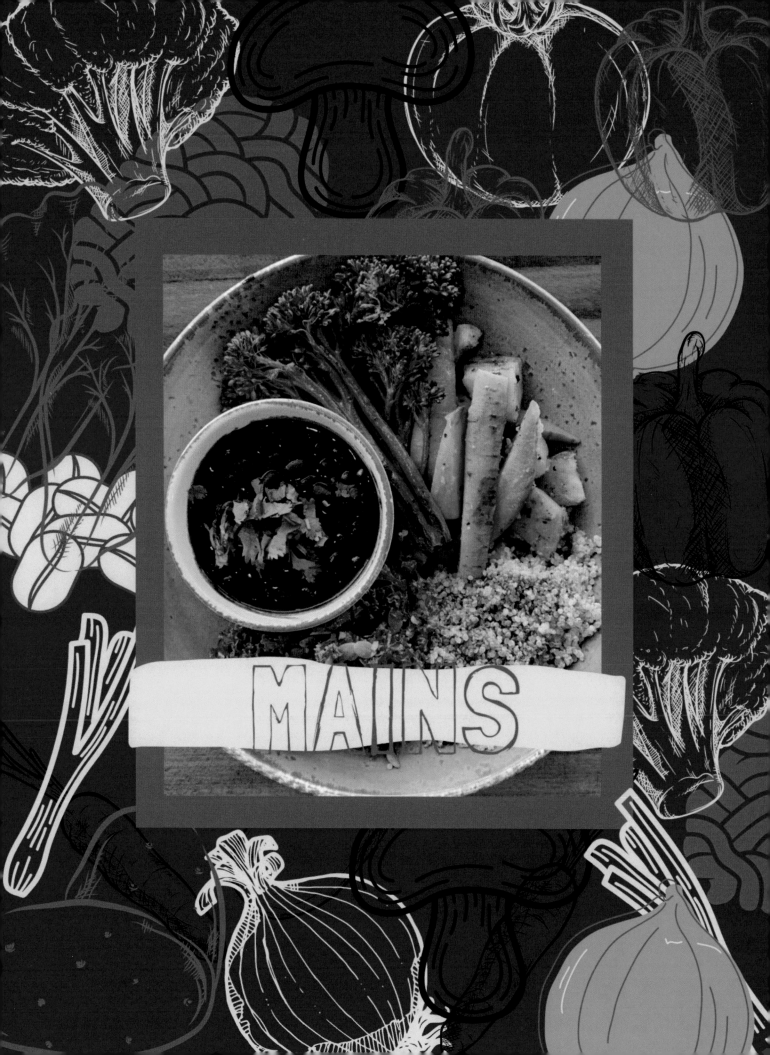

MAINS

PIZZA IDEAS

Alfredo Pizza w/ broccoli, mushrooms, red onions

Pita Pizzas

Thai Pizza w/peanut sauce, chickpeas, shredded carrots, zukes

Vegan Parmesean w/cashews, nutritional yeast, garlic powder

Caprese Pizza w/ vegan mozzarella, sliced tomatoes, basil, Italian seaoning

BBQ Pizza w/ cauliflower, garlic sauce, bacon tempeh, green onions

English Muffin Pizzas

Spinach & artichoke

Deep Dish Pizza

Sauteed peppers, mushrooms and onions

Greek Pizza w/ hummus, chickpeas, olives, red onions, basil

Taco Pizza w/ sundried tomatoes & walnut taco meat

Chickpea Flour Pizza with roasted sweet potatoes, hummus

Dessert Pizza w/ pie crust, fruit, coconut, nuts

Bagel Pizzas

Butternut squash, apples and pecans

Roasted sweet potato, corn, jalapenos

Pizza Bar - Make Your Own

Breakfast Pizza w/ vegan egg, vegan cheese sauce, tempeh bacon

French Bread Pizza

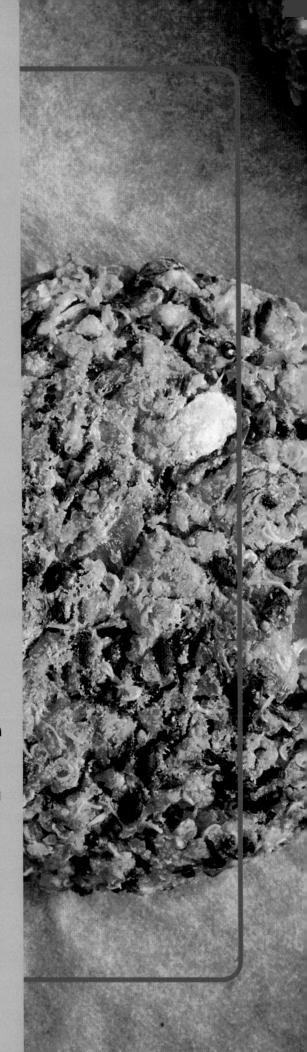

SPICY QUINOA & BEAN BURGERS

1/2 cup uncooked quinoa

1 can black beans, rinsed and drained

1–2 jalapeño or chipotle peppers diced

1/2 tsp each: onion powder, chili powder, cumin, smoked paprika

vegan egg: 1 Tbs ground chia seed mixed with 3 Tbs water (let set 10 min)

1 tsp salt

1/4 cup panko or breadcrumbs

2 cloves smashed garlic

Cook quinoa according to package directions and allow to cool. Make vegan egg.

Combine black beans, quinoa, peppers, garlic and spices, in a food processor. Pulse just a few times, enough to make the mixture sticky and well-mixed but not completely pureed. Okay to have chunks of bean still intact.

Add vegan egg and panko: Transfer mixture to a large bowl. Mix egg and panko. Form into 4 thick burgers.

Add burgers to hot frying pan and cook for a few minutes on each side, flipping carefully to keep them intact, until they are golden brown and crispy on the outside. Or you can bake at 375°F for 10-15 minutes on each side.

toast
1 block of tempeh, sliced thinly
4 Tbs maple syrup
4 Tbs coconut aminos
1/2 tsp liquid smoke
2-3 leaves of romaine lettuce/other favorite green
1/2 thinly sliced tomato
favorite mustard
optional sesame seeds

BLT

Place tempeh in water in a frying pan to soften for about 5 minutes, drain water. In small bowl, mix sauce while softening the tempeh. Brown tempeh on both sides in frying pan, pour 1/2 sauce mix on tempeh and cook 1 minute, then flip and add the rest of the sauce, cook another minute until a little crisp.

For Your Masterpiece:
Arrange tempeh bacon, lettuce, and tomato on one side of sliced toasted bread. Add desired amount of mustard. Place other half of toasted bread on top.

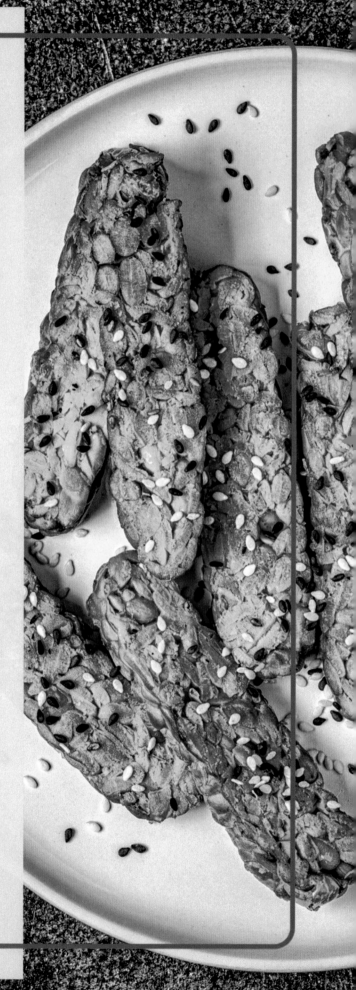

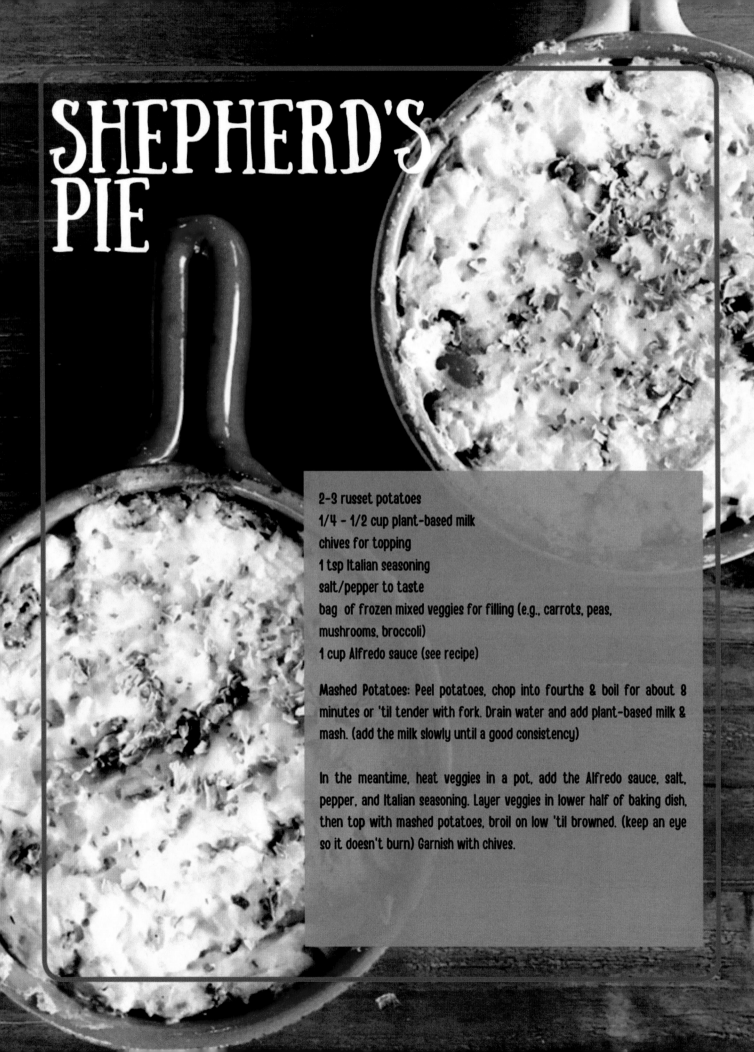

SHEPHERD'S PIE

2-3 russet potatoes
1/4 - 1/2 cup plant-based milk
chives for topping
1 tsp Italian seasoning
salt/pepper to taste
bag of frozen mixed veggies for filling (e.g., carrots, peas, mushrooms, broccoli)
1 cup Alfredo sauce (see recipe)

Mashed Potatoes: Peel potatoes, chop into fourths & boil for about 8 minutes or 'til tender with fork. Drain water and add plant-based milk & mash. (add the milk slowly until a good consistency)

In the meantime, heat veggies in a pot, add the Alfredo sauce, salt, pepper, and Italian seasoning. Layer veggies in lower half of baking dish, then top with mashed potatoes, broil on low 'til browned. (keep an eye so it doesn't burn) Garnish with chives.

SOUTHWEST BOWL

1 cup cooked rice or wild rice (sub quinoa optional)

1/2 cup black beans (see seasoning from Rustic Bowl)

1 1/2 cups mixed greens, chopped

1/2 bell pepper, diced

pico de gallo (see recipe)

1/4 cup roasted corn

1 radish, sliced

1-2 Tbs sour cream (see recipe)

cilantro, handful, chopped

guacamole (see recipe)

lime cubed

To construct your bowl: Place items in sections. Start with a scoop of rice, then beans, then fill the other half with fresh greens, add small section of radish, top the remaining greens with bell peppers, pico de gallo, and corn. Drizzle on the sour cream, add a dollop of guacamole and a sprinkle of cilantro and wedge of lime.

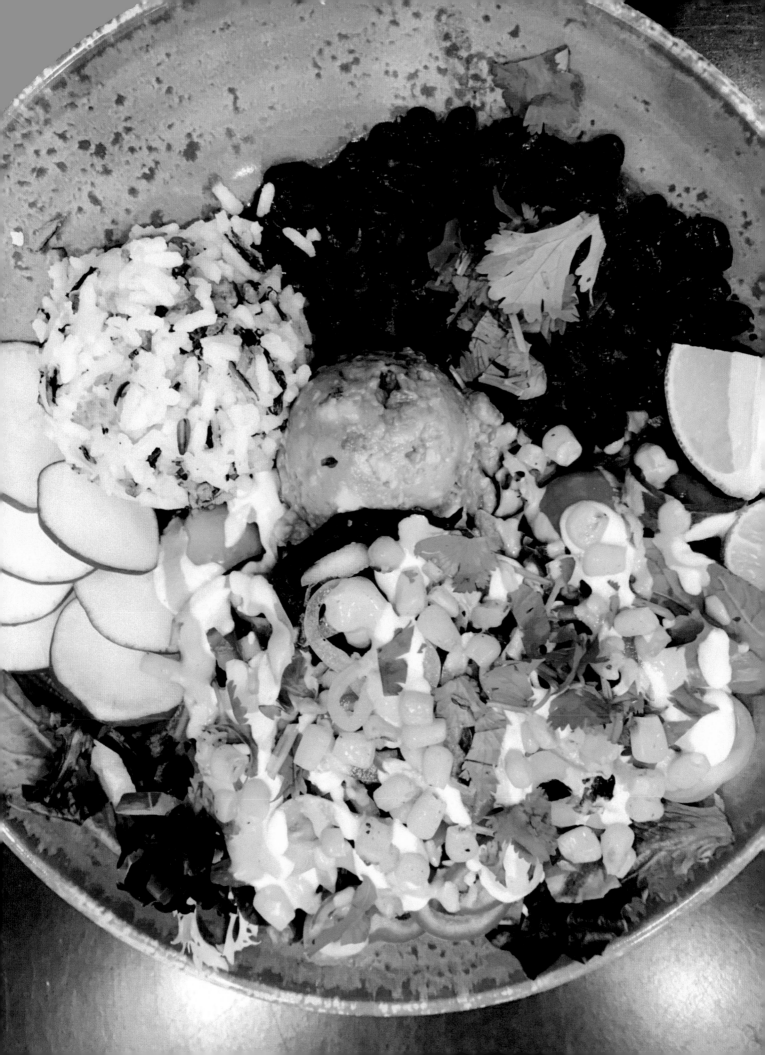

RUSTIC BOWL

Massage kale with lemon juice. Cook and season all ingredients separately. Combine in bowl, top with glaze, seeds, and sprouts.

Suggested seasoning for black beans: 1/4 tsp of chili powder, onion powder, garlic powder, cumin, oregano, salt, 1/4 C chopped onion, cilantro, 2 bay leaves, squeeze of lime.

Toppings: Balsamic glaze (see recipe), pumpkin seeds, pinch of broccoli sprouts

½ cup black beans, rinsed and drained

1-2 cups of kale, chopped

1 medium roasted russet potato or sweet potato

1 cup quinoa, cooked

chopped ½ cup broccolini, steamed and chopped

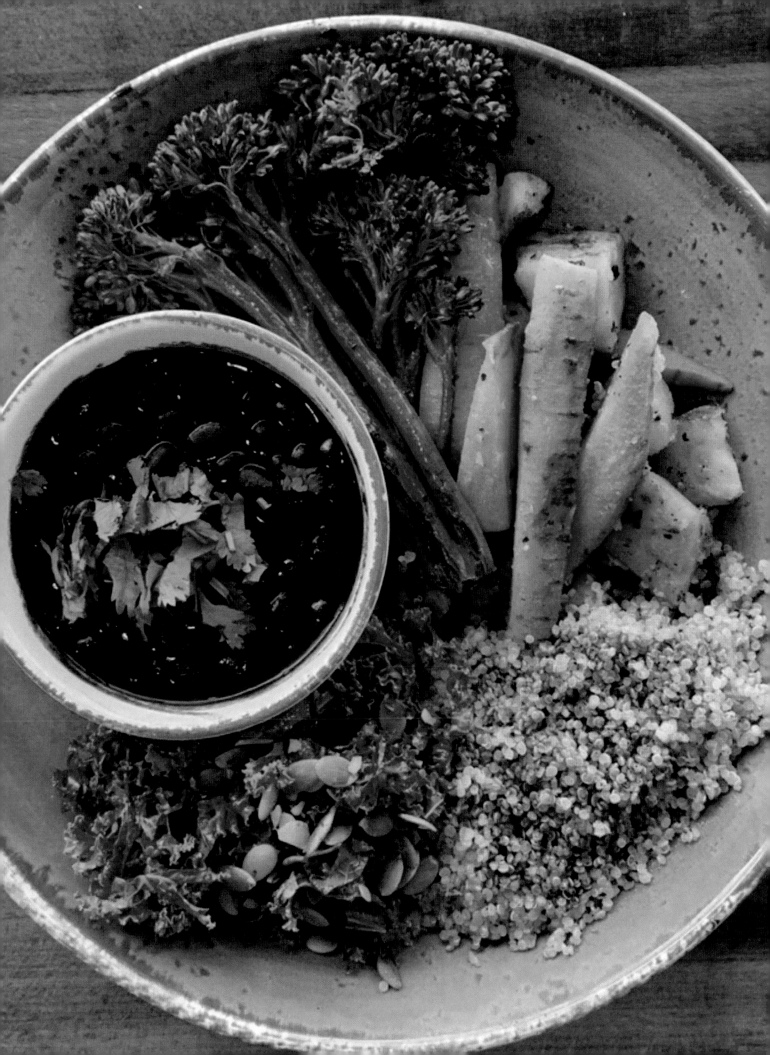

GRILLED VEGETABLES OVER PASTA OR SALAD

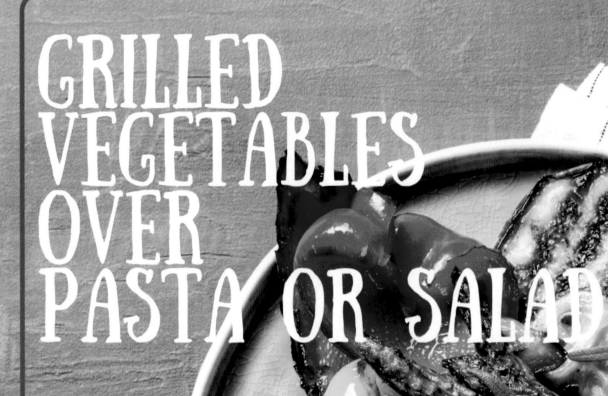

1 eggplant, sliced into thin steaks

small tomatoes whole

asparagus

rosemary

veggie broth to toss

kosher salt & pepper

Italian seasoning blend

bell peppers, thick slices

zucchini, sliced

Slice vegetables the same thickness (1/3"-1/2"), toss with veggie broth, sprinkle over Italian seasoning, kosher salt, and pepper. Grill on the BBQ at 350-450°F flipping halfway through. Start with the bell peppers, then add the rest of the veggies after 5 minutes so they are done at the same time. Bell peppers take about 10-12 minutes, the others take about 5-8 minutes. Serve over cooked pasta with Alfredo sauce or over a bed of greens with avocado.

MARINATED TOFU W/ RICE AND SAUTEED VEGGIES

1 package firm tofu, drained, diced

1/4 cup water

2 Tbs tamari sauce

1 Tbs apple cider vinegar

1 Tbs maple syrup

1 tsp garlic powder

pinch of cayenne powder

1 tsp cornstarch

2 cups of cooked white basmati rice

1 package of frozen stir-fried veggies

1 cup shredded cabbage

Extra tamari sauce

Mix all ingredients, except tofu and veggies, in a bowl. Then add the tofu and let sit in refrigerator covered for 1 hour. Remove the tofu, saving the liquid. Sauté the tofu in a non-stick frying pan until golden brown. Add water if it begins to stick. Add the cornstarch to the saved marinade and whisk until well mixed. Add the mixture to the tofu pan and heat until thickened. Heat stir fried veggies according to package. Add shredded cabbage to tofu pan along with heated veggies. Heat until all combined and warmed. Serve over rice with additional tamari sauce if desired.

TEXMEX TOFU CUBES

Extra firm organic tofu x 2 packages
2 Tbs vinegar
1 Tbs water or more as needed for a thick sauce
1 tsp cumin
1 tsp chili powder
1 tsp garlic powder
¾ tsp salt
½ tsp chipotle powder
½ tsp smoked paprika

Preheat oven to 400°F   Cut tofu into small cubes and place in a bowl that has a spill-proof lid or use a large baggie. Mix other ingredients together in a small bowl, pour over the tofu, seal the container and shake to coat the tofu cubes. Place coated tofu on a parchment-lined baking sheet.   Bake for 15 minutes.   For extra crispy, broil an additional 2-4 minutes.

Serve in a corn tortilla with guacamole and arugula or taco toppings such as guacamole, pico de gallo, and sour cream.

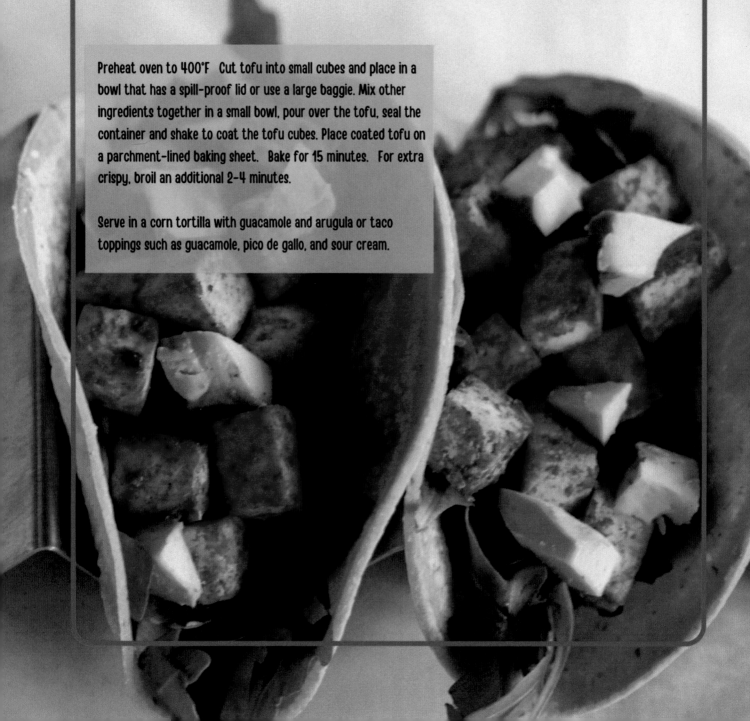

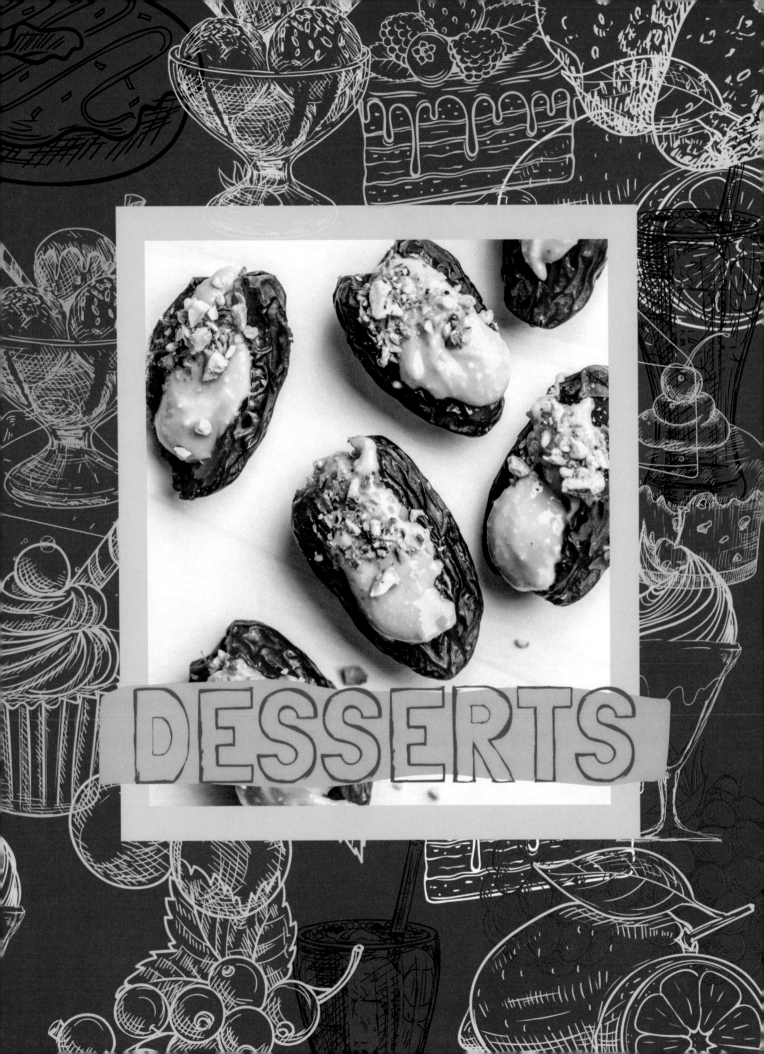

DESSERTS

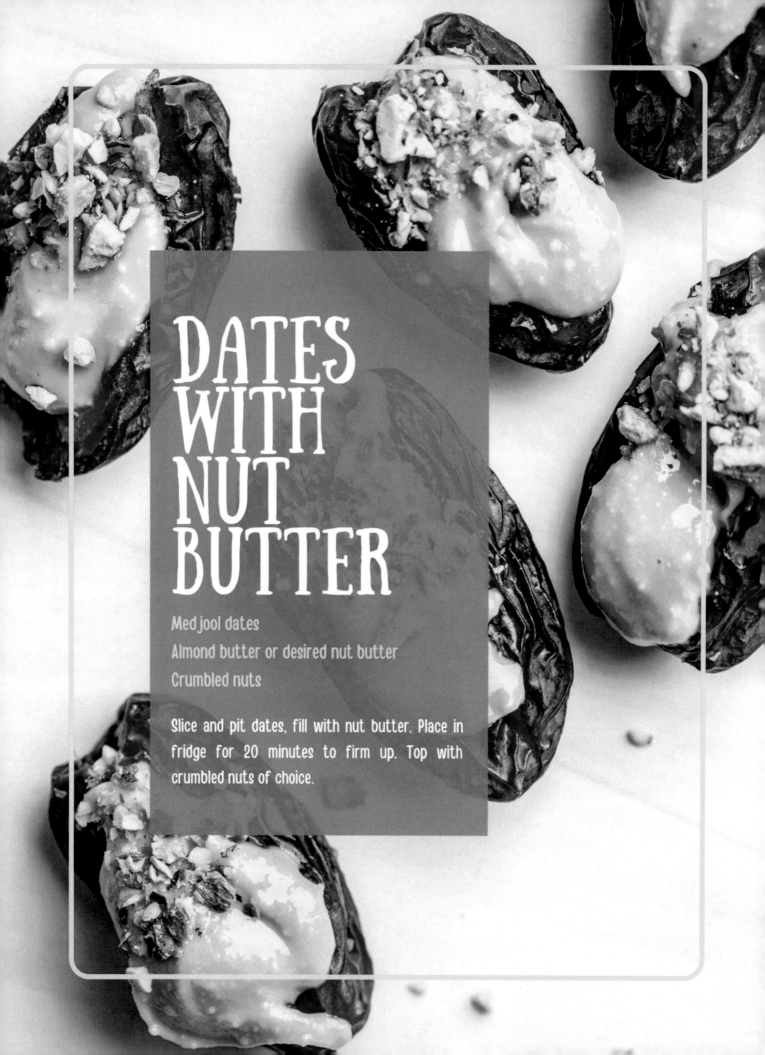

DATES WITH NUT BUTTER

Medjool dates

Almond butter or desired nut butter

Crumbled nuts

Slice and pit dates, fill with nut butter. Place in fridge for 20 minutes to firm up. Top with crumbled nuts of choice.

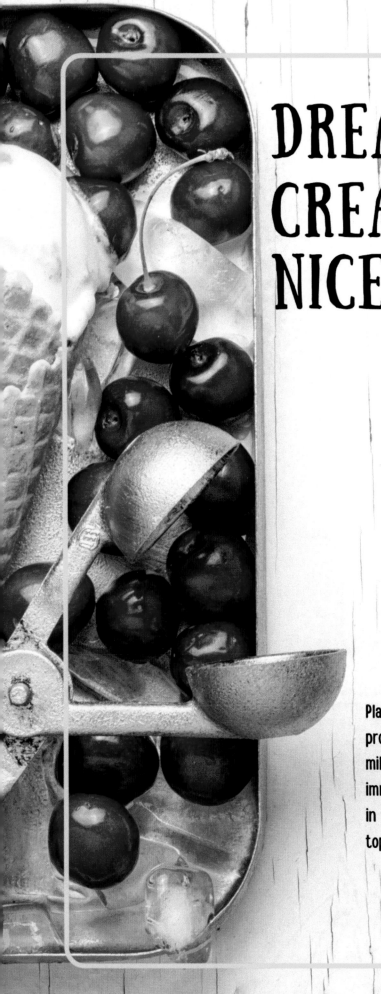

DREAMY SWEET CREAMY CHERRY NICE CREAM

4-5 medium frozen bananas

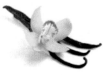

1/4 tsp vanilla

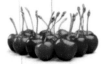

1 cup frozen, pitted cherries

2-4 tsp plant-based milk (optional)

Place cherries, bananas, and vanilla into food processor and process until completely smooth. Add milk if a thinner consistency is desired. Eat immediately or place in air-tight container and store in freezer. Serve with cacao nibs, nuts, or granola on top.

Chapter Fifteen

RESOURCES & SOURCES

●●●

20 Top Resources You Can Use

1. *The China Study* by Dr. Colin Campbell
2. *Eat to Live* by Dr. Joel Fuhrman
3. *Prevent and Reverse Heart Disease* by Dr. Caldwell Esselstyn Jr.
4. *The Cheese Trap* by Dr. Neal Barnard
5. *The Pleasure Trap* by Dr. Dean Ornish
6. *The Starch Solution* by Dr. John & Mary McDougall
7. *My Beef with Meat* by Rip Esselstyn
8. *How Not to Die* by Dr. Michael Greger
9. *Goodbye Lupus* by Dr. Brooke Goldner
10. *Vegan Burgers & Burritos* by Sophia DeSantis
11. *Thug Kitchen: Eat Like You Give A F**k* by Thug Kitchen
12. *Vegan Richa's Indian Kitchen* by Richa Hingle

13. *Forks Over Knives* produced by Lee Fulkerson

14. *The Game Changers* produced by James Cameron

15. *What the Health* produced by Kip Anderson & Keegan Kuhn

16. *Cowspiracy* produced by Kip Anderson & Keegan Kuhn

17. *Eating You Alive* produced by Paul David Kennamer Jr.

18. www.forksoverknives.com

19. www.pcrm.org

20. www.nutritionfacts.org

SOURCES

Chapter One

1. Krebs-Smith SM, Guenther PM, Subar AF, Kirkpatrick SI, Dodd KW. Americans do not meet federal dietary recommendations. *J Nutr.* 2010, 140(10): 1832–1838.
2. https://www.cdc.gov/chronicdisease/about/costs. Accessed January 6, 2021

Chapter Two

1. Mozaffarian D, Aro A, Willett WC. Health effects of trans-fatty acids: experimental and observational evidence. *Eur J Clin Nutr.* 2009, 63(2): S5-21.
2. Ghafoorunissa, G. Role of trans fatty acids in health and challenges to their reduction in Indian foods. *Asia Pac J Clin Nutr.* 2008, 17(1): 212-5.
3. Gillman MW, Cupples LA, Gagnon D, Millen BE, Ellison RC, Castelli WP. Margarine intake and subsequent coronary heart disease in men. *Epidemiology.* 1997, 8(2): 144-9.
4. Willett WC, Stampfer MJ, Manson JE, Colditz GA, Speizer FE, Rosner BA, Sampson LA, Hennekens CH. Intake of trans fatty acids and risk of coronary heart disease among women. *Lancet.* 1993, 341(8845): 581-5.
5. https://Federalregister.gov/documents/2015/06/17/2015-14883/final-determination-regarding-partially-hydrogenated-oil. Accessed January 6, 2021

6. https://nutritionfacts.org/2019/08/27/vegans-should-consider-taking-dha-supplements/. Accessed January 6, 2021

7. Swanson D, Block R, Mousa SA. Omega-3 fatty acids EPA and DHA: Health benefits throughout life. *Adv Nutr.* 2012, 3(1): 1–7.

8. Neff LM, Culiner J, Cunningham-Rundles S, Seidman C, Meehan D, Maturi J, Wittkowski KM, Levine B, Breslow JL. Algal docosahexaenoic acid affects plasma lipoprotein particle size distribution in overweight and obese adults. *J Nutr.* 2011, 141(2): 207-13.

9. Simplício PS, Mediano MFF, Silva GMS, Brito PD, Cardoso CSA, Almeida CD, Sangenis LHC, Pinheiro RO, Hasslocher-Moreno AM, Alvarenga PE, Brasil A, Sousa, AS. Omega-3 supplementation on inflammatory markers in patients with chronic Chagas cardiomyopathy: A randomized clinical study. *Nutr J.* 2017, 16: 36.

10. Tan ZS, Harris WS, Beiser AS, Au R, Himali JJ, Debette S, Pikula A, Decari C, Wolf PA, Vasan RS, Robins SJ, Seshadri S. Red blood cell ω-3 fatty acid levels and markers of accelerated brain aging. *Neurology.* 2012, 78(9): 658-64.

11. Hunter P. The inflammation theory of disease: The growing realization that chronic inflammation is crucial in many diseases opens new avenues for treatment. *EMBO Rep.* 2012 Nov, 13(11): 968–970.

12. Esselstyn CB Jr., Gendy G, Doyle J, Golubic M, Roizen MF. A way to reverse CAD? *J Fam Pract.* 2014, 63(7): 356-364.

13. Esselstyn C. Resolving the coronary artery disease epidemic through plant-based nutrition. *Prevent Card.* 2001, 4: 171–177.

14. https://www.pcrm.org/good-nutrition/nutrition-information/protein. Accessed January 6, 2021.

15. Berrazaga I, Micard V, Gueugneau M, Walrand S. The role of the anabolic properties of plant- versus animal-based protein sources in supporting muscle mass maintenance: A critical review. *Nutrients*. 2019, 11(8): 1825.

16. Naghshi S, Sadeghi O, Willett WC, Esmaillzadeh A. Dietary intake of total, animal, and plant proteins and risk of all cause, cardiovascular, and cancer mortality: Systematic review and dose-response meta-analysis of prospective cohort studies. *BMJ*. 2020, 370: 2412-2429.

17. Song M, Fung TT, Hu FB, Willett WC, Longo VD, Chan AT, Giovannucci EL. Association of animal and plant protein intake with all-cause and cause-specific mortality. *JAMA Intern Med*. 2016, 176(10): 1453-1463.

18. Aune D, Giovannucci E, Boffetta P, Fadnes LT, Keum N, Norat T, Greenwood DC, Riboli E, Vatten LJ, Tonstad S. Fruit and vegetable intake and the risk of cardiovascular disease, total cancer and all-cause mortality-a systematic review and dose-response meta-analysis of prospective studies. *Int J Epidemiol*. 2017, February 22.

19. https://www.cdc.gov/heartdisease/facts.html. Accessed January 6, 2021.

20. https://www.cancer.org/research/cancer-facts-statistics/all-cancer-facts-figures/cancer-facts-figures-2020.html. Accessed January 6, 2021.

21. https://www.cdc.gov/diabetes/pdfs/data/statistics/national-diabetes-statistics-report.pdf. Accessed January 6, 2021.

22. https://www.who.int/news-room/fact-sheets/detail/cancer. Accessed January 6, 2021.

23. https://www.who.int/health-topics/cardiovascular-diseases#tab=tab_1/. Accessed January 6, 2021.

24. https://www.who.int/news-room/fact-sheets/detail/diabetes#tab=tab_1. Accessed January 6, 2021.

25. https://www.worldobesity.org/about/about-obesity/prevalence-of-obesity. Accessed January 6, 2021.

Chapter Three

1. Bradbury KE, Murphy N, Key TJ. Diet and colorectal cancer in UK Biobank: A prospective study. *Int J Epidemiol.* 2020, 49(1): 246-258.

2. De Jauregi DR-F, Evans CEL, Jones P, Greenwood DC, Hancock N, Cade JE. Common dietary patterns and risk of cancers of the colon and rectum: Analysis from the United Kingdom Women's Cohort Study (UKWCS). *Int J Cancer.* 2018, 143(4): 773-781. https://www.who.int/mediacentre/news/statements/2015/processed-meat-cancer/en/. Accessed January 6, 2021.

3. Seah JYH, Gay GMW, Su J, Tai E-S, Yuan J-M, Koh W-P, Ong, CN, van Dam, RM. Consumption of red meat, but not cooking oils high in polyunsaturated fat, is associated with higher arachidonic acid status in Singapore Chinese adults. *Nutrients.* 2017, 9(101): 1-14.

4. Wang X, Lin X, Ouyang YY,Liu, J, Zhao G, Pan A, Hu FB. Red and processed meat consumption and mortality: dose-response meta-analysis of prospective cohort studies. *Public Health Nutr.* 2016, 19(5): 893-905.

5. https://www.nih.gov/news-events/nih-research-matters/eating-red-meat-daily-triples-heart-disease-related-chemical. Accessed January 6, 2021.

6. Micha R, Michas G, Mozaffarian D. Unprocessed red and processed meats and risk of coronary artery disease and type 2 diabetes—An updated review of the evidence. *Curr Atheroscler Rep*. 2012, 14(6): 515–524.

7. Taylor EF, Burley VJ, Greenwood DC, Cade JE. Meat consumption and risk of breast cancer in the UK women's cohort study. *British Journal of Cancer*. 2007, 96: 1139–1146.

8. Linos E, Willett WC, Cho E, Colditz G, Frazier LA. Red meat consumption during adolescence among premenopausal women and risk of breast cancer. *Cancer Epidemiol Biomarkers Prev*. 2008, 17(8): 2146–51.

9. Zhang S,Wang Q, He J. Intake of red and processed meat and risk of renal cell carcinoma: a meta-analysis of observational studies. *Oncotarget*. 2017, 8(44): 77942–77956.

10. Singh PN, Sabaté J, Fraser GE. Does low meat consumption increase life expectancy in humans? *Am J Clin Nutr*. 2003, 78(suppl): 526S–32S.

11. Esposito K, Giugliano F, Maiorino MI, Giugliano D. Dietary factors, Mediterranean diet and erectile dysfunction. *Review J Sex Med*. 2010, 7(7): 2338-45.

12. Salas-Huetos A, Bulló M, Salas-Salvadó J. Dietary patterns, foods and nutrients in male fertility parameters and fecundability: A systematic review of observational studies. *Human Reproduction Update*. 2017, 23(4): 371–389.

13. Wang Y, Beydoun MA. Meat consumption is associated with obesity and central obesity among US adults. *Int J Obes (Lond)*. 2009, 33(6): 621-628.

14. Barnard ND, Goldman DM, Loomis JF, Kahleova H, Levin SM, Neabore S, Batts TC Plant-based diets for cardiovascular safety and performance in endurance sports. *Nutrients*. 2019, 11(1): 130.

15. Zhang Y, Yang Y, Xie M-S, Ding X, Li H, Liu Z-C, Peng S-F. Is meat consumption associated with depression? A meta-analysis of observational studies. *BMC Psychiatry*. 2017, 17(409).

16. Pereira da Silva AP, Costa DC, Aguiar L, Matos A, Gil A, Gorjão-Clara J, Polónia J, Bicho M. Impact on longevity of genetic cardiovascular risk and lifestyle including red meat consumption. *Oxidative Medicine and Cellular Longevity*. 2020. https://doi.org/10.1155/2020/1305413. Accessed January 6, 2021.

17. Qin L, Xu J, Wang P, Tong J, Hoshi K. Milk consumption is a risk factor for prostate cancer in Western countries: Evidence from cohort studies. *Asia Pac J Clin Nutr*. 2007, 16: 467–476.

18. Campbell TC, Campbell TM. *The China study: the most comprehensive study of nutrition ever conducted and the startling implications for diet, weight loss, and long-term health*. 2016, (Revised and expanded ed.). *Ben Bella Books*.

19. https://www.pcrm.org/good-nutrition/nutrition-information/health-concerns-about-dairy. Accessed January 6, 2021.

20. Zhong VW, Van Horn L, Cornelis MC, Wilkins JT, Ning H, Carnethon MR, Greenland P, Mentz RJ, Tucker KL, Zhao L, Norwood AF, Lloyd-Jones DM, Allen NB. Associations of dietary cholesterol or egg consumption with incident cardiovascular disease and mortality. *JAMA*. 2019, 321(11): 1081-1095.

21. Chia SJ, McRae JL, Kukuljan S, Woodford K, Elliott RB, Swinburn B, Dwyer KM. A1 beta-casein milk protein and other environmental predisposing factors for type 1 diabetes. *Nutr Diabetes*. 2017, 7(5): e274.

22. Hoppe C, Mølgaard C, Juul A, Michaelsen KF. High intakes of skimmed milk, but not meat, increase serum IGF-I and IGFBP-3 in eight-year-old boys. *Eur J Clin Nutr*. 2004, 58(9): 1211-6.

23. Hussain SM, Cicuttini FM, Giles GG, Graves SE, Wluka AE, Wang Y. Association between dairy product consumption and incidence of total hip arthroplasty for osteoarthritis. *J Rheumatol*. 2017, 44(7): 1066-1070.

24. Song Y, Chavarro JE, Cao Y, Qui W, Mucci L, Sesso HD, Stampfer MJ, Giovannucci E, Pollak M, Liu S, Ma J. Whole milk intake is associated with prostate cancer-specific mortality among U.S. male physicians. *J Nutr*. 2013, 143: 189-196.

25. Chan JM, Stampfer MJ, Ma J, Gann PH, Gaziano JM, Giovannucci E. Dairy products, calcium, and prostate cancer risk in the Physicians' Health Study. *Am J Clin Nutr*. 2001, 74: 549-554.

26. Go Y, Chung M, Park Y. Dietary patterns for women with triple-negative breast cancer and dense breasts. *Nutrition and Cancer*. 2016, 68(8): 1281-1288.

27. Melnik BC. Evidence for acne promoting effects of milk and other effects of milk and other insulinotropic dairy products. *Nestle Nutr. Inst. Workshop Ser Pediatr Program*. 2011, 67: 131-145.

28. http://www.medicalnewstoday.com/articles/322593. Accessed January 6, 2021.

29. Severance EG, Dickerson FB, Halling M, Krovogorsky B, Haile L, Yang S, Stallings CR, Origoni AE, Bossis I, Xiao J, Dupont D. Haasnoot W, Yolken RH. Subunit and whole molecule specificity of the anti-bovine casein immune response in recent onset psychosis and schizophrenia. *Schizophrenia Research*. 2010, 118(1-3): 240-247.

30. https://www.pcrm.org/news/blog/five-frightful-facts-about-cheese. Accessed January 6, 2021.

31. Zhong VW, Van Horn L, Cornelis MC, Wilkins JT, Ning H, Carnethon MR, Greenland P, Mentz RJ, Tucker KL, Zhao L, Norwood AF, Lloyd-Jones DM, Allen NB. Associations of dietary cholesterol or egg consumption with incident cardiovascular disease and mortality. *JAMA*. 2019, 321(11): 1081-1095.

32. Ramaekers VT, Sequeria JM, Blau N, Quadros EV. 2008. A milk-free diet down regulates folate receptor autoimmunity in cerebral folate deficiency syndrome. *Dev. Med Child Neuro.* 2008, 50(5) 346-352.

33. Jiang W, Ju C, Jiang H, Zhang D. Dairy foods intake and risk of Parkinson's Disease: a dose-response meta-analysis of p prospective cohort studies. *Eur. J. Epidemiol.* 2014, 29(9): 613-9.

34. Juhl CR, Helle K. Bergholdt M, Miller IB, Gregor BE, Jørgen J, Kanters K, Ellervik, C. Dairy intake and acne vulgaris: A systematic review and meta-analysis of 78,529 children, adolescents, and young adults. *Nutrients.* 2018, 10(8): 1049.

Chapter Four

1. Mugiea SM, Benning MA, Di Lorenzo C. Epidemiology of constipation in children and adults: A systematic review. *Best Practice & Research Clinical Gastroenterology.* 2011, 25(1): 3-181.

2. Sanchez MIP, Bercik P. Epidemiology and burden of chronic constipation. *Can J Gastroenterol.* 2011, 25(Suppl B): 11B–15B.

3. https://www.caloriesecrets.net/how-much-fibre-should-we-eat-in-a-day/ Accessed on January 6, 2021.

4. Barnard ND. The effects of a low-fat, plant-based dietary intervention on body weight, metabolism, and insulin sensitivity. *Am J Med.* 2005, 118(9): 991–7.

5. Tabung F, Steck SE, Su LJ, Mohler JL, Fontham ETH, Bensen JT, Hebert JR, Zhang H, Arab L. Intake of grains and dietary fiber and prostate cancer aggressiveness by race. *Prostate Cancer*. 2012, 323296. Published online 2012 Nov 13. doi: 10.1155/2012/323296PMCID: PMC3503404PMID: 23213538. Accessed January 6, 2021.

6. Pereira MA, O'Reilly E, Augustsson K, Fraser E, Goldbourt U, Heitmann BL, Hallmans G, Knekt P, Liu S, Pietinen P, Spiegelman D, Stevens J, Virtamo J,Walter C. Willett WC, Ascherio A. Dietary fiber and risk of coronary heart disease a pooled analysis of cohort studies. *Arch Intern Med*. 2004, 164(4): 370-376.

7. McRae MP. Dietary fiber intake and type 2 diabetes mellitus: An umbrella review of meta-analyses. *J Chiropr Med*. 2018, 17(1): 44–53.

8. de Jauregui DR-F, Evans CEL, Jones P, Greenwood DC, Hancock N, Cade JE. Common dietary patterns and risk of cancers of the colon and rectum: Analysis from the United Kingdom Women's Cohort Study (UKWCS). *International Journal of Cancer*. 2018, 143(4): 773-781.

9. Fuchs CS, Giovannucci EL, Colditz GA, Hunter DJ, Stampfer MJ, Rosner B, Speizer FE, Willet WC. Dietary fiber and the risk of colorectal cancer and adenoma in women. *N Engl J Med*. 1999, 340(3): 169-176.

10. Bagga D, Ashley JM, Geffrey SP, Wang, HJ, Barnard RJ, Koerenman S, Heber D. Effects of a very low fat, high fiber diet on serum hormones and menstrual function: Implications for breast cancer prevention. *Cancer*. 1995, 76: 2491-2496.

11. Soler M, Bosetti C, Franceschi S, Negri E, Zambon P, Talamini R, Conti E, La Vecchia C. Fiber intake and the risk of oral, pharyngeal and esophageal cancer. *Int J Cancer*. 2001, 91(3): 283-287.

12. https://my.clevelandclinic.org/health/diseases/10352-diverticular-disease. Accessed January 6, 2021.

13. https://www.arthritis.org/health-wellness/healthy-living/nutrition/anti-inflammatory/increasing-fiber. Accessed January 6, 2021.

14. Myhrstad MCW, Tunsjo H, Charnock C, Telle-Hansen VH. Dietary fiber, gut microbiota and metabolic regulation – current states in human randomized trials. *Nutrients*. 2020, 12(3): 859.

15. Park Y, Subar AF, Hollenbeck A, Schatzkin A. Dietary fiber intake and mortality in the NIH-AARP diet and health study. *Arch Intern Med*. 2011, 171(12): 1061–1068.

Chapter Five

1. Buetner D, Skemp S. The Blue Zones: Lessons from the world's longest lived. *Am J Lifestyle Med*. 2016, 10(5): 318-321.

2. Ganesan K, Xu B. Polyphenol-rich dry common beans (Phaseolus vulgaris L.) and their health benefits. *Int J Mol Sci*. 2017, 18(11): 2331.

3. Barnard ND, Bush AI, Ceccarelli A, Cooper J, Celeste A, de Jager K, Erickson I, Fraser G, Kesler S, Levin SM, Lucey B, Morris MC, Squitti R. Dietary and lifestyle guidelines for the prevention of Alzheimer's disease. *Neurobiology of Aging*. 2014, 35 (Supplement 2): S74-S78.

4. https://www.aicr.org/cancer-prevention/food-facts/dry-beans-and-peas-legumes/. Accessed January 7, 2021.

5. https://www.amymyersmd.com/article/benefits-greens/. Accessed January 7, 2021.

6. Mano R, Ishida A, Ohya Y, Todoriki H, Takishita S. Dietary intervention with Okinawan vegetables increased circulating endothelial progenitor cells in healthy young women. *J Atherosclerosis*. 2009, 204(2): 544-8.

7. Pollock RL. The effect of green leafy and cruciferous vegetable intake on the incidence of cardiovascular disease: A meta-analysis. *JRSM Cardiovasc Dis*. 2016, 5: 204.

8. https://www.nia.nih.gov/news/leafy-greens-linked-slower-age-related-cognitive-decline. Accessed January 7, 2021.

9. https://www.sciencedaily.com/releases/2018/10/181019100558.htm. Accessed January 7, 2021.

10. https://thebeet.com/what-to-eat-for-better-sex-dr-caldwell-esselstyn-on-how-to-eat-now/. Accessed January 7, 2021.

Chapter Six

1. https://www.who.int/news-room/fact-sheets/detail/obesity-and-overweight. Accessed January 7, 2021.

2. https://hsph.harvard.edu/obesity-prevention-source/obesity-consequences/economic. Accessed January 7, 2021.

3. https://www.who.int/health-topics/cardiovascular-diseases/#tab=tab_1. Accessed January 7, 2021.

4. Rajendran P, Rengarajan T, Thangavel J, Nishigaki Y, Sakthisekaran D, Sethi G, Nishigaki I. The vascular endothelium and human diseases. *Int J Biol Sci*. 2013, 9(10): 1057–1069.

5. https://www.cancer.org/research/cancer-facts-statistics/all-cancer-facts-figures/cancer-facts-figures-2020.html. Accessed January 7, 2021.

6. https://www.who.int/news-room/fact-sheets/detail/cancer. Accessed January 7, 2021.

7. https://www.cdc.gov/diabetes/pdfs/data/statistics/national-diabetes-statistics-report.pdf. Accessed January 7, 2021.

8. https://www.who.int/news-room/fact-sheets/detail/diabetes. Accessed January 7, 2021.

9. https://nationalstemcellfoundation.org/glossary/autoimmune-disease/. Accessed January 7, 2021.

10. Procaccini C, Carbone F, Galgani M, La Rocca C, De Rosa V, Cassano S, Matarese G. Obesity and susceptibility to autoimmune diseases. *Expert Rev Clin Immunol*. 2011, 7(3): 287–294.

11. https://www.who.int/news-room/fact-sheets/detail/dementia. Accessed January 7, 2021.

12. Okereke O, Rosner B, Kim D, Kang JH, Cook NR, Manson JE, Buring JE, Willett WC, Grodstein F. Dietary fat types and 4-year cognitive change in community-dwelling older women. *Ann. Neurol*. 2012, 72(1): 124-34.

13. https://www.osteoporosis.org.au/sites/default/files/files/WOD16-report-PRESS-FINAL.pdf. Accessed January 7, 2021.

14. Office of the Surgeon General (US). Bone health and osteoporosis: A report of the Surgeon General. Rockville (MD). 2004, 4, The Frequency of Bone Disease. https://www.ncbi.nlm.nih.gov/books/NBK45515/. Accessed January 7, 2021.

15. McCabe LD, Martin BR, McCabe GP, Johnston CC, Weaver CM, Peacock M. Dairy intakes affect bone density in the elderly. *Clinical Trial Am J Clin Nutr*. 2004, 80(4): 1066-74.

16. Feskanich D, Willett WC, Stampfer MJ, Colditz GA. Milk, dietary calcium, and bone fractures in women: A 12-year prospective study. *American Journal of Public Health*. 1997, 87(6): 992-997.

17. Michaëlsson K, Wolk A, Langenskiöld S, Basu S, Warensjö E, Lemming, Melhus H, Byberg L. Milk intake and risk of mortality and fractures in women and men: cohort studies and observational study. *BMJ*. 2014, 28: 349.

18. https://www.health.harvard.edu/diseases-and-conditions/glycemic-index-and-glycemic-load-for-100-foods. Accessed January 7, 2021.

CHAPTER EIGHT

1. Garner B, Lally P, Wardle J. Making health habitual: The psychology of "habit-formation" and general practice. *British Journal of General Practice*. 2012, 62(605): 664-666.

2. Lally P, Va Jaarsveld CHM, Potts HWW, Wardle J. How are habits formed: Modeling habit formation in the real world. *Eur. J. Soc. Psychol.* 2010, 40: 998-1009.

Made in the USA
Monee, IL
28 May 2021